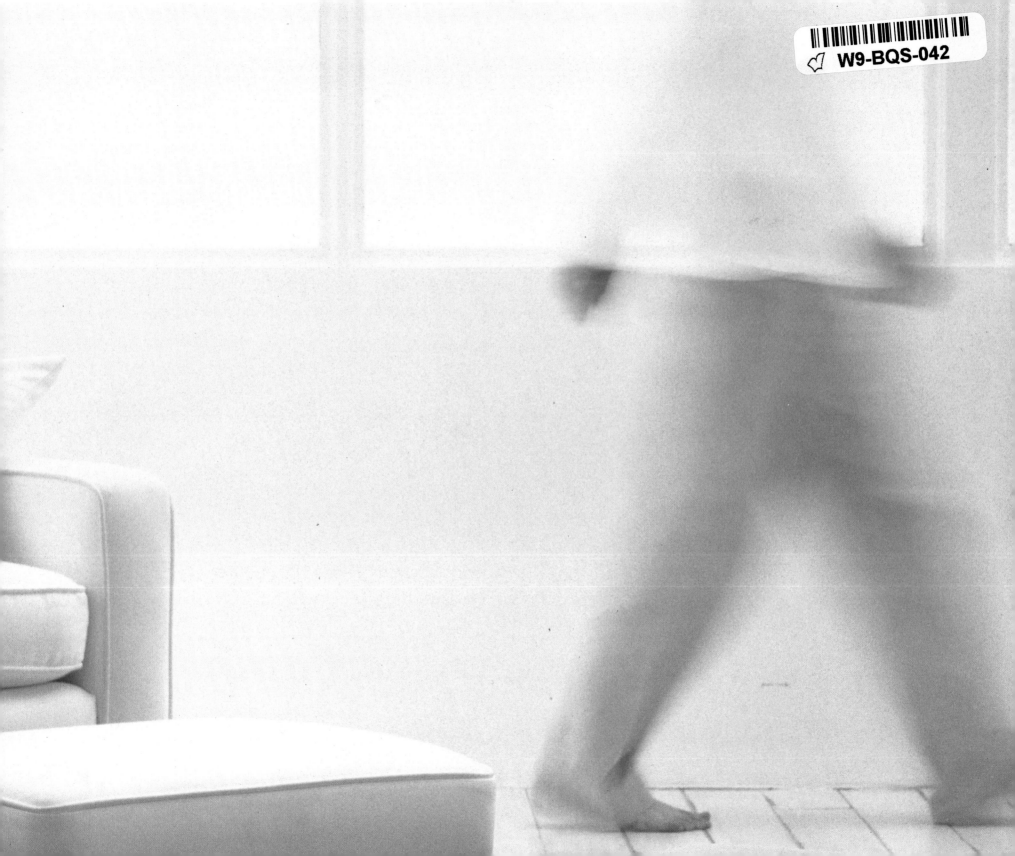

Yoga Life

Discover Health and Well-Being, All Day, Every Day

Lorna Lee Malcolm

DUNCAN BAIRD PUBLISHERS

LONDON

To Winston, Darren, Michael, Patrick and Nick – the adult men in my life that I love. To Louise, Sonji and Denise – the women that I love. To Conrad, Alexander, Zakari and Theodore – my four gorgeous nephews who fill me totally with love, inspiration and laughter. To my family.

Yoga Life

Lorna Lee Malcolm

This edition published in the United Kingdom and Ireland in 2005 by
Duncan Baird Publishers Ltd
Sixth Floor, Castle House
75–76 Wells Street, London W1T 3QH

Conceived, created and designed by Duncan Baird Publishers
Copyright © Duncan Baird Publishers 2001
Text copyright © Duncan Baird Publishers 2001
For copyright of photographs see page 164, which is to be regarded as an extension of this copyright

Managing Editor: Judy Barratt
Consultant Editor: Kesta Desmond
Editor: Richard Emerson
Managing Designer: Manisha Patel
Designer: Rachel Cross
Model photography: Matthew Ward
Picture research: Julia Ruxton

British Library Cataloguing-in-Publication Data:
A catalogue record for this book is available from the British Library

10 9 8 7 6 5 4 3 2 1

ISBN-10: 1-84483-124-8   ISBN-13: 9-781844-831241

Typeset in Helvetica Condensed, Helvetica Light and Son-Kern
Colour reproduction by Colourscan, Singapore
Printed by Imago, Singapore

Publisher's note

Before following any advice or exercise in this book, we recommend that you ask your doctor whether it is suitable for you, especially if you suffer from any health disorders or special conditions. The publishers, the author and the photographer cannot accept responsibility for any injuries or damage incurred as a result of following the exercises in this book, or of using any of the therapeutic methods described or mentioned here.

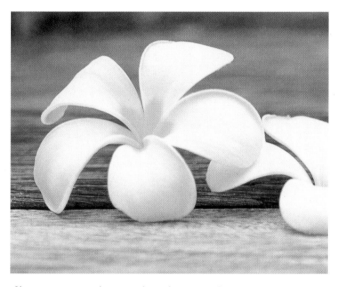

"Harmony in eating and resting, in sleeping and waking:
perfection in all you do. This is the path to peace."

The Bhagavad Gita

CONTENTS

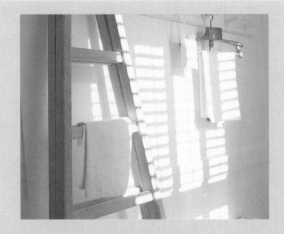
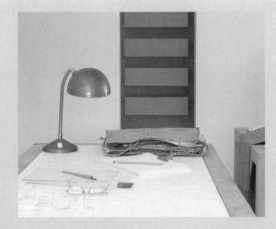
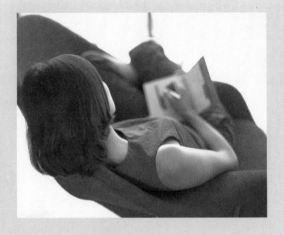

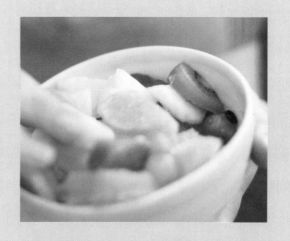
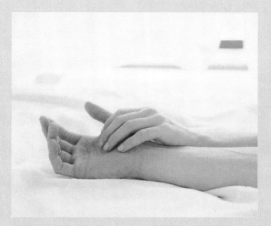
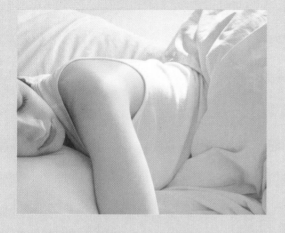

HOW TO USE THIS BOOK

The aim of *Yoga Life* is simple – to help you have a great day. But the advice it offers may enable you to achieve much more than that. It can show you how to enhance your physical and emotional health and well-being, and bring order and control into your life and have a healthy, fulfilling lifestyle.

The emphasis is firmly on the practical. Throughout *Yoga Life* you'll find a variety of easy – yet effective – techniques to try at home. Most of the information comes from traditional Eastern disciplines and therapies, such as yoga, t'ai chi, and acupressure. These are centuries-old ways of improving your health, pacifying your mind, relaxing your body, tapping into your inner nature and aligning your mind, body and spirit. But all have been tailored to make them relevant to a contemporary Western way of life.

Yoga Life is divided into six chapters, each one representing an aspect of a typical day. The first chapter, Waking, explains how to start the morning in a mood of tranquillity and optimism and prepare for the day ahead. Chapter 2, Working, helps you to work productively and overcome problems such as poor concentration, stress and muscular tension. Chapter 3, Relaxing, looks at the art of mental, physical and spiritual relaxation. Chapter 4, Eating and Drinking, shows you how to optimize your health and well-being through your diet. Chapter 5, Loving, tackles relationships and how to enhance them through touch, massage, movement and by cultivating feelings of love and compassion. The final chapter, Sleeping, teaches you how to wind down from the day and prepare your mind and body for deep, satisfying rest.

Interspersed throughout the book are special double-page spreads overlaid with translucent paper designed to generate a unique mood. These pages feature fully illustrated step-by-step sequences of exercises or postures that enable you to reach a goal – such as achieving calm, relaxation, mental clarity, even intimacy – through physical movement. To gain maximum benefits, aim to practise one or more of these sequences daily.

All of the exercises in *Yoga Life* are simple and safe to do and should not cause you pain or physical strain. If any movement or posture makes you feel dizzy, strange or uncomfortable, stop the exercise and sit quietly until you feel better. If you have an ongoing health problem – such as a disorder of the heart, lungs, spine or joints – check with your doctor or other relevant health-care specialist before you try any of these exercises.

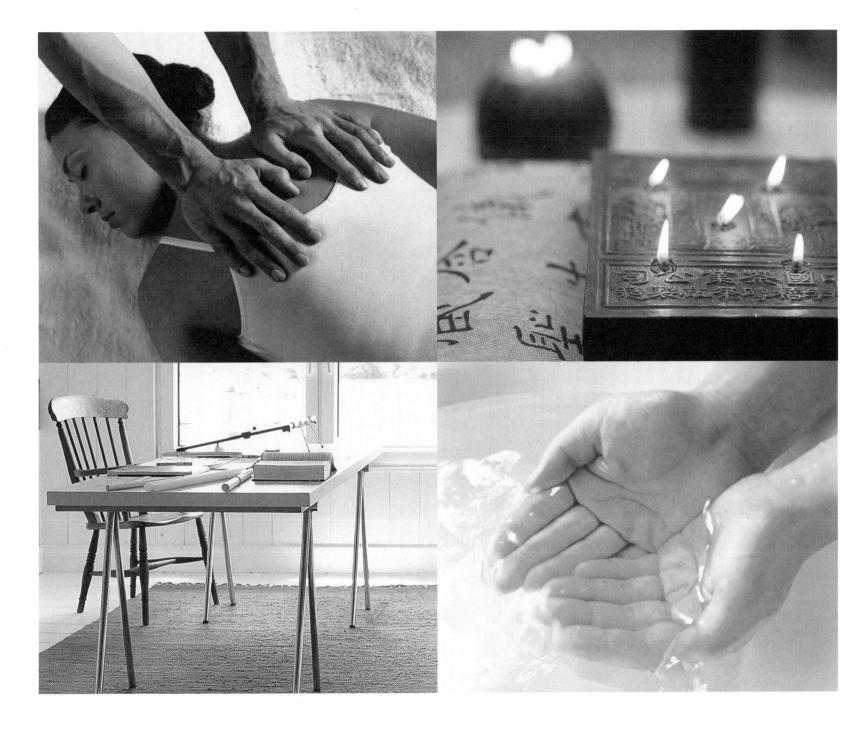

INTRODUCTION

Hi there. I have three sincere wishes for you. The first is that the style and content of this book encourages you to reflect on your life. All too often, in today's hectic world, we do not give ourselves time to reflect and, instead, let our mind and emotions become detached from our physical being. We miss so much because we are not aware of the moment. Before we know it, time has moved on and we are left wondering where it went. Juggling the many aspects of our day, suffering a constant build-up of stress and leaving little time for self can all detract from our quality of life.

When we live reactively, we do not allow ourselves time to be a conscious participant and enjoy our experiences to the full. We lose connection with our inner self and find ourselves surviving rather than truly living, always trying to reach a point or achieve a goal rather than enjoying the journey. I hope this book will highlight the importance of changing your lifestyle and working healthy practices into your day, in a way that suits you.

I would ask you, as you read this book, to reflect on all aspects of your life, as well as reflecting on yourself and who you are currently. Consider how well you know yourself and whether you do justice to the person you are? Are you truly aware of what makes you stressed and, in turn, what enables you to release that stress and relax? How well do you balance work, home/family and social life? A balanced life is not about dealing with every-thing equally but about what is appropriate for you, paying due respect and consideration to all the elements that make up your world.

My second wish would be that having taken time to reflect, you then take action on anything that you feel you want to change. To use myself as an example, I was a practising solicitor for nine years. Toward the end of that period, I found the job had ceased to be satisfying. I was working with people with whom I had nothing in common and in a building that, through its design and lack of natural light, deflated my mood every time I entered. On a few occasions, it got to the stage where I would get up and get ready, travel to work, then immediately get the bus home and call in sick.

I knew I could not continue in this way. It made me stop, take a step back and re-assess my life. I decided that, despite the money I was earning, I needed more – a change of working environment that would not come about by just changing jobs. I needed to move on, to do something I would enjoy. I decided to make what had been my hobby, my profession. My career is now health and fitness. I lecture, present to and educate other instructors all over the world, consult for Reebok, write and teach regular classes each week. It was a nerve-racking decision and I took time making it.

Having researched and planned as much as I could, I took the plunge and have not regretted the decision for a second. I can't believe I now get paid for doing something I love! This shows how important it is to be proactive; to acknowledge any aspect about your life that you are unhappy or dissatisfied with, and aim to change it. Research, plan step by step and then take action – because you owe it to yourself to be happy and fulfilled.

This leads me on to my final wish. We often hear that "life is not a rehearsal", and "you only get one chance in this world". Even if you believe in reincarnation, you should still live your life to the full. Being of good health, mentally as well as physically, can only enhance that. Studies show that regular exercise (not necessarily of the frantic kind) and increased physical activity can help reduce the risk of certain diseases. It may prevent or, if pre-existing, manage various conditions such as high blood pressure, coronary heart disease, osteoporosis and certain types of diabetes, to name but a few. It can also alleviate anxiety and mild depression and generally enhance one's mental state, self-confidence and self-esteem.

Living life to the full should result in a happy, expressive "you", with a calmness of spirit and an acknowledgment of the importance of love. Happiness comes from having a positive outlook and approach; by seeing problems as challenges rather than obstacles. Calmness of spirit should flow from knowing who you are, what you're working toward and would like to achieve and also being aware of, and open to, enjoying the journey. With your increased awareness and value of life, I hope you will not want to waste time and energy bearing grudges or ill feeling toward others.

May I suggest that you use this book for reference and revisit certain chapters as their content becomes relevant to particular periods, situations or emotions. Use the book to recharge flagging batteries and to remind yourself, from time to time, of any commitment you have made to yourself and your chosen lifestyle. Happy reading and happy living!

Lorna

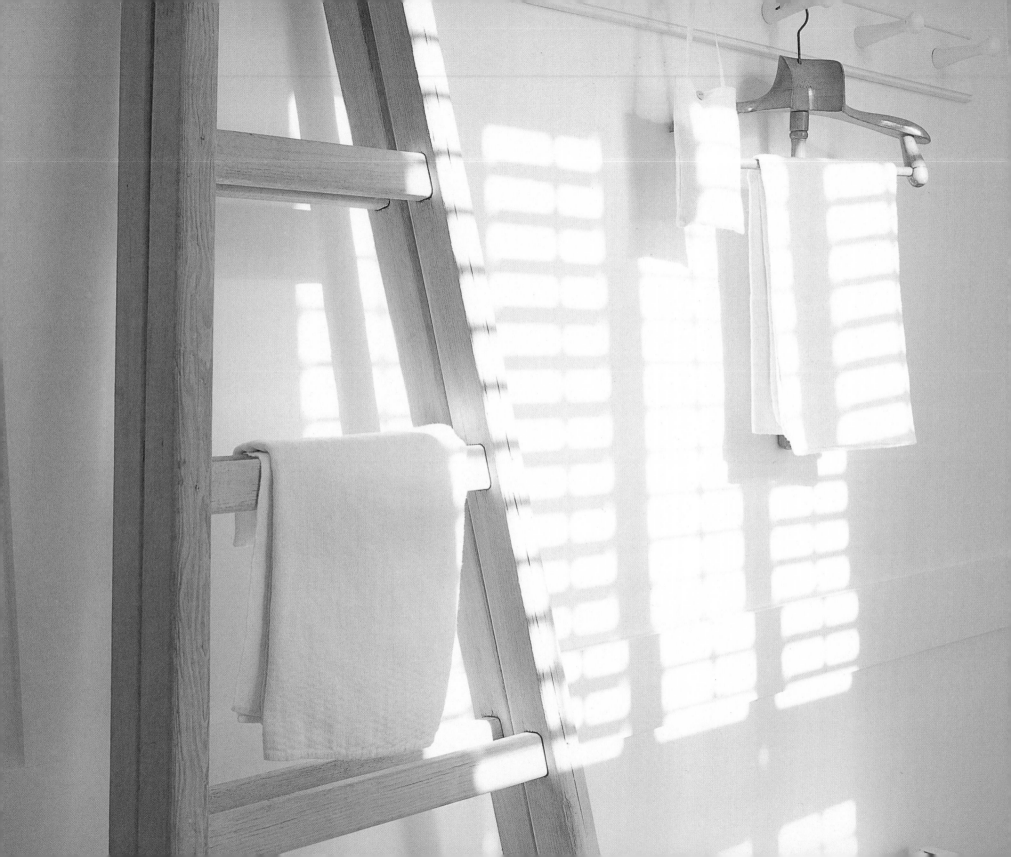

WAKING

How you feel in the morning can greatly influence the way in which the rest of your day unfolds. If you feel invigorated and in a positive frame of mind, these feelings will permeate through your day and help you to deal with life's ups and downs with energy, equanimity, good humour and a sense of purpose.

This chapter presents a wide range of exercises and techniques that you can use to prepare yourself for the day ahead: affirmations to create a positive mood, stretches to invigorate your body, t'ai chi and qigong to harness your energy, and breathing and meditation to focus your mind.

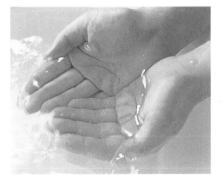

A POSITIVE START

When you first open your eyes you should greet the new day feeling positive, refreshed and free from cares. Yet if you wake to the prospect of a rushed and stressful day, you are being burdened by negative thoughts from the very moment you are conscious. Positive affirmations help to rid you of these negative thoughts by "overwriting" them with positive ones. Whereas techniques such as meditation bring mental peace by stilling *all* mental activity, positive affirmations have a calming influence on the mind by training it to develop a happier outlook.

Negative thoughts are far from innocuous. They can have a damaging effect on both your physical and emotional health. A constant barrage of worries, anxieties, pessimistic thoughts and self-criticism steadily erodes self-esteem, making you feel less happy, less at peace and even downright disillusioned with life. Over time, this can leave you vulnerable to health problems such as depression, chronic fatigue, headaches, palpitations, digestive problems and viral infections, such as colds and 'flu.

Positive affirmations work because the unconscious mind faithfully records every emotional response you have – good or bad. If you tell yourself repeatedly that you are confident, happy and peaceful, these messages are logged in your unconscious and will be reflected in your day-to-day moods and actions. If, on the other hand, your unconscious mind receives only negative messages, such as "I can't cope" or "I'm useless", these nagging thoughts can very quickly become self-fulfilling prophecies.

Practise your affirmations as soon as you get up in the morning. The events of the day have not yet begun and even a busy mind is receptive to suggestions at this time. You don't have to sit down in a quiet room or close your eyes (although you can do this if you find it helpful). You can do your affirmations still lying in bed, while getting dressed, or in the shower – in fact anywhere at all. Some people find that their affirmations are reinforced if they do them while looking in the mirror. Whether you say them out loud or silently to yourself is entirely up to you.

Tailor your affirmations to suit the needs and challenges you expect to be facing on that particular day. For example, if one day you're feeling nervous, your affirmation could be: "I am strong and confident and I can handle everything that today might throw at me." It's important to keep the language of your affirmations positive, so, for example, if your affirmation is "I don't feel tired",

This day finds me happy and content. I am ready
to start the day with optimism and an open mind.

The world is a wonderful place filled with
kind people and loving actions.

I forgive myself for any mistakes I made yesterday.

My breath is my constant companion. When I feel anxious
I breathe deeply and I start to feel calmer.

Today I accept myself and others and see the good
and the valuable in us all.

I accept whatever I am feeling today. I can let my feelings
come and go and be open to whatever experience is next.

Every day is full of miracles.

recast this as "I feel rested, awake and ready to face the day." Aim to construct your affirmations in the present tense. This makes them feel like firmly held beliefs that are real and immediate instead of mere possibilities still waiting to happen.

When you practise affirmations, remember that your unconscious mind responds best to one or two short, uncluttered statements that are repeated frequently and persistently. It also registers images better than words alone, so use visualization techniques to reinforce your belief. For example, if your affirmation is: "I stay calm in the face of stress and difficulty", visualize yourself as the captain of a boat with your hands on the tiller. Imagine yourself steering a straight and steady course through the waves, even when they become rough.

On the left are a few general examples of positive affirmations that you can use each morning to put you in the right frame of mind for the day ahead. You can say them as written, adapt them to your own needs or substitute your own beliefs. As you think about the words you're saying, invest each one with emotion. The unconscious absorbs these messages uncritically, so if you say them often enough they become reality.

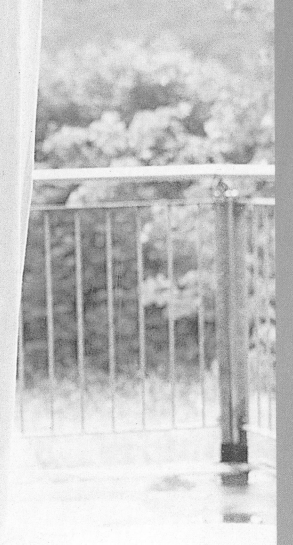

MORNING STRETCH

After the inactivity of sleep it feels great to wake up your body by giving it a good, long stretch. The following morning stretch sequence is designed to ease the stiffness of sleep and counter-act the stagnant energy of a night spent in bed. It is a version of a classic yoga practice, "salute to the sun", and is a perfect way to wake the body. It stretches the spine, removes stiffness from the muscles and stimulates blood flow to the brain – the ideal sequence of postures to energize you at the start of the day.

In Hindu belief, dawn is the time of day when the air is rich in life-force energy (known as *prana*). The synchrony of breath and movement in these postures helps to enhance the flow of this energy around the body. As you do the whole sequence, breathe deeply through your nose, inhaling during the upward lifting movements and exhaling during the downward movements.

Keep your movements smooth and let each one flow easily into the next. Stretch the muscles all over your body. Think of the way that cats and dogs stretch after a nap – they push their front legs forward and lengthen the entire spine. Step 4 imitates this lengthening. Practise the whole sequence at least six times and alternate the leading leg in step 5 each time.

MORNING SEQUENCE

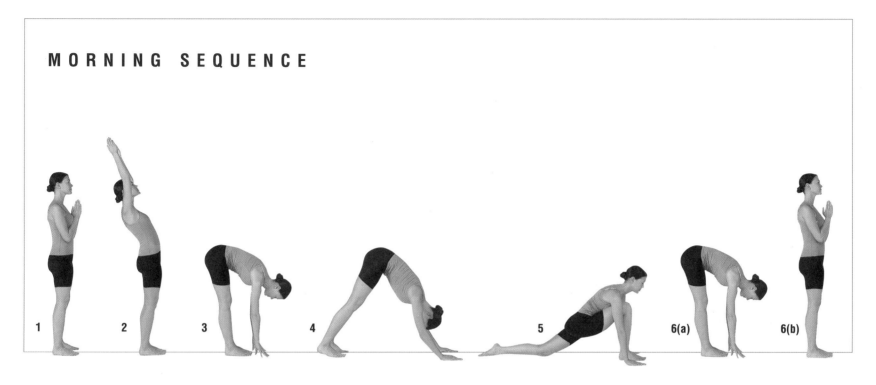

1   **Start in a standing posture with your feet slightly apart and your hands together as if in prayer.**

2   **Inhale as you stretch your arms over your head and lean back slightly. Keep your head in line with your arms. Stretch your fingers.**

3   **Exhale and fold forward at your hips, keeping your back flat. Rest your hands on the ground, bending your knees as necessary.**

4   **Exhale and step your feet back. Push your hips back and up and press your heels down to the ground. Draw up your thigh muscles. Keep your back and head in a straight line and your abdominal muscles pulled up toward your spine.**

5   **Inhale and step your right foot forward between your hands to come into a deep lunge with your left knee on the floor. Look ahead.**

6   **(a) Exhale and lift your hips high and step your left foot forward to meet the right foot. Bend your knees to keep your hands on the ground. (b) Inhale and return to the standing position by hinging at your hips and keeping your back flat. Raise your arms over your head and then exhale and bring your hands back into the prayer position.**

INVIGORATE YOUR BODY

HARNESS PURE ENERGY

CALM YOUR THOUGHTS

"Harmony in eating and resting, in sleeping and waking: perfection in all you do. This is the path to peace." The Bhagavad Gita

T'AI CHI ENERGIZER

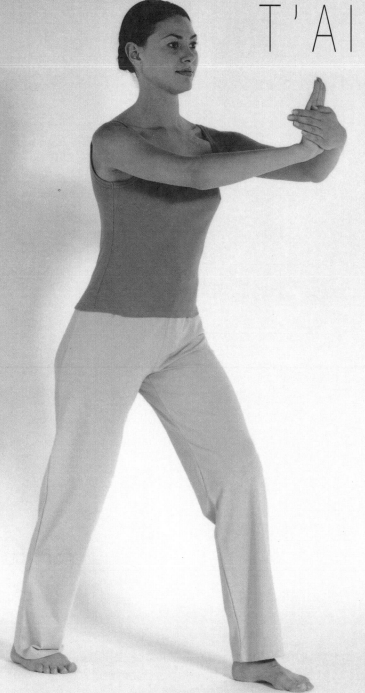

A traditional way to start the day in China is to practise the beautifully fluid movements of t'ai chi in the open air. T'ai chi is thought to have originated in 12th-century China as a form of martial art, like a softer version of kung fu. Although you are unlikely to use t'ai chi for self-defence, the state of relaxed alertness that t'ai chi fosters is an excellent way to prepare yourself for the day ahead.

T'ai chi offers many physical and emotional benefits: it strengthens muscles, encourages the flow of life-force energy (*qi* or *chi* – equivalent to the Hindu *prana*) through the body and fosters regular breathing, which helps you to react calmly and intelligently to challenging situations.

The main practice in t'ai chi is known as the "form", which consists of a set sequence of postures (between 24 and 108) that are performed as seamless flowing movements. The best way to learn the form is from an experienced t'ai chi teacher who is knowledgeable about all aspects of t'ai chi, including its spiritual and philosophical sides. However, the following t'ai chi exercise (known as pushing and pulling) is easily learned. It aims to balance *yin* and *yang* – in Taoist philosophy, the two equal but opposing forces that control the universe. Practise the pushing and pulling exercise when you rise in the morning, before you have your breakfast. It can help to relax and focus the mind and enhance strength, balance, flexibility and posture. Wear comfortable, loose-fitting clothes and concentrate on making your movements and breathing slow, smooth and regular.

PUSHING AND PULLING

Stand with your feet shoulder-width apart, arms by your sides and inhale. Raise your left arm slightly and bend it at the elbow so that it is parallel with the ground. Your palm should face the centre of your chest. Place your right palm against your left palm with your right elbow pointing down. Step your left foot forward. Use your right palm to push your left palm beyond your left foot (opposite) as you exhale. Then, press your right hand in toward your chest with your left hand. Inhale and return your weight to your right foot (right). Finish off by standing with your feet parallel and shoulder-width apart and open your arms to the sides with elbows bent and palms facing forward. Exhale. Do this whole sequence five times and then repeat on the other side.

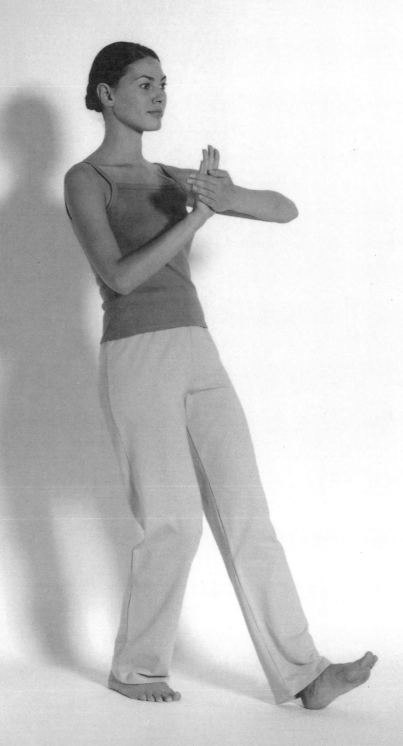

QIGONG ENERGIZERS

The two qigong exercises on the following pages can help you to tune into your natural flow of energy and harness it at the start of the day. Qigong (pronounced "chee goong") is one of the pillars of traditional Chinese medicine, along with t'ai chi, herbalism and acupuncture. *Qi* (or *chi*) is the life-force energy that flows through the body and gives us life and vitality. *Gong* means work, so qigong means "energy for work". Qigong is an internal process that relies upon mental focus and concentration. By sensing your internal *qi* you can nurture it and increase its strength, thereby enhancing your physical, emotional and spiritual well-being. *Qi* can be a difficult concept to understand – as well as being at odds with orthodox Western beliefs – so you may find it difficult to sense your internal energy flow, at least at first. Give yourself time and don't be self-critical. Not everyone finds it easy.

In Chinese philosophy, the seat of the body's energy is in the lower abdomen – an area known as the *dan tien* – three finger

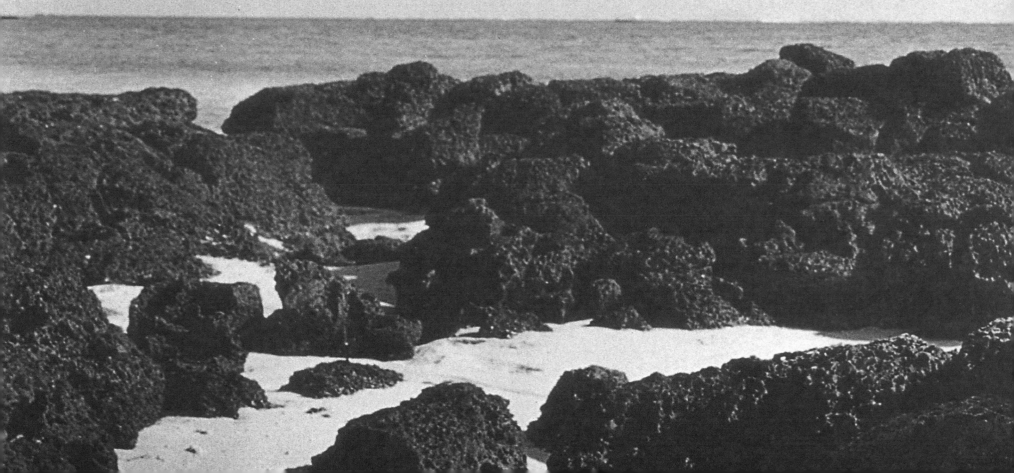

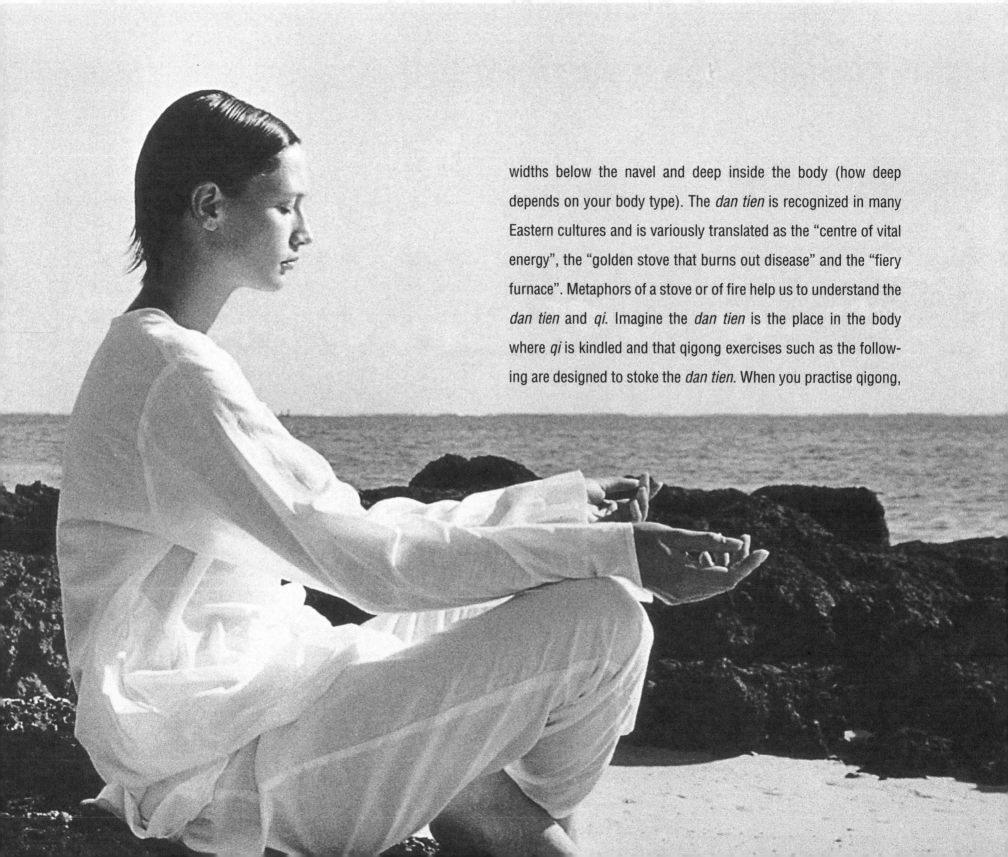

widths below the navel and deep inside the body (how deep depends on your body type). The *dan tien* is recognized in many Eastern cultures and is variously translated as the "centre of vital energy", the "golden stove that burns out disease" and the "fiery furnace". Metaphors of a stove or of fire help us to understand the *dan tien* and *qi*. Imagine the *dan tien* is the place in the body where *qi* is kindled and that qigong exercises such as the following are designed to stoke the *dan tien*. When you practise qigong,

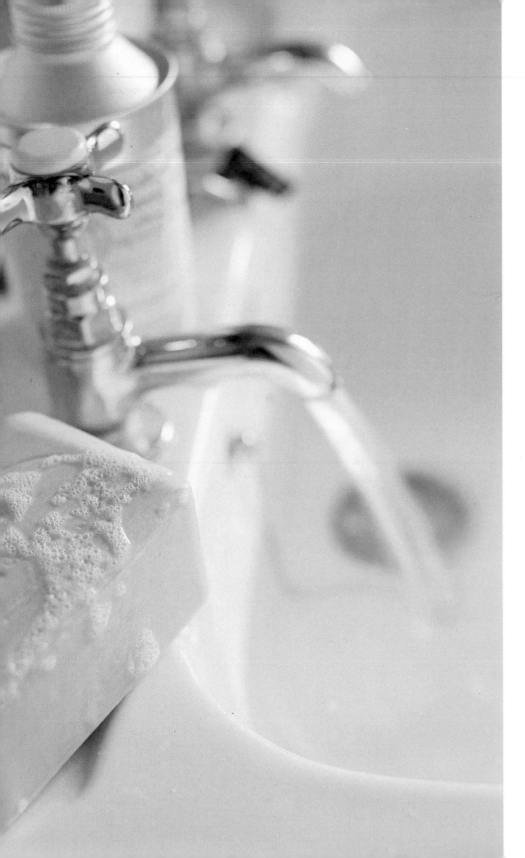

it's important to breathe into the *dan tien* by taking your breath down deeply into your abdomen. The first exercise is called "sensing a ball of energy" and helps you to feel the energy that emanates from the *dan tien*. As you practise steps 2 and 4, visualize this ball of energy. Focus on the sensations between your palms and in your abdomen. Once you are accustomed to this exercise, you should start to feel a sensation of warmth or tingling in your palms and fingers – or you may feel as though you are really holding a ball.

The second exercise is called "rotating a ball of energy" and builds on the intuitive skills you have learned from the first exercise. By rotating the ball both mentally and physically you can increase the *qi* within your *dan tien*. This is an ideal way to cultivate energy at the start of the day. You can also use it to revive yourself later on in the day if you feel tired or sluggish.

SENSING A BALL OF ENERGY

Stand in the *Wu Chi* position (see page 72). Bend your arms and bring your palms to face each other in front of your lower abdomen. Imagine a small ball of energy between your hands coming from your abdomen. Stay like this for two minutes. Imagine the ball of energy is growing bigger and pushing your hands apart (below, right). Allow the space between your palms to grow to roughly shoulder-width. Stay like this for one minute. Imagine the ball of energy is contracting and pulling your hands together again. Bring your palms back in front of your abdomen.

Once the ball of energy is fully contracted, cup your hands around it and visualize it condensing into a tiny bright light. As it does so, press one palm against your lower abdomen with the other palm on top. Imagine the light vanishing deep into your abdomen. Take your hand away.

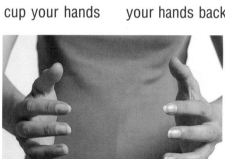

ROTATING A BALL OF ENERGY

Stand in the *Wu Chi* position. Bend your elbows slightly and bring your hands – fingertips nearly touching and palms facing up – to your lower abdomen. Sense the power emanating from the ball of energy in your lower abdomen. Stay here for two minutes and imagine the energy filling your palms. Imagine your palms are supporting the bottom of the energy ball. Slowly bring your hands

around the front of the ball so that your palms are facing in toward your abdomen. Imagine you are rotating the energy ball. Rotate your hands until they are resting on top of the ball of energy, at the level of your ribs.

Leading with your thumbs, bring your hands behind the ball. Imagine you are creating space in your lower abdomen. Bring your hands back underneath the ball and twist them so they are back to the starting position again. Repeat this rotation exercise 20 times. At the end of your last rotation, imagine the energy ball condensing into a point of light inside your abdomen. Press your palms, one on top of the other, on your lower abdomen.

After doing these qigong exercises, your hands will be charged with fresh *qi*. Rather than allowing this to disperse, you can use it to refresh yourself – rub your hands together and then cup your hands over your eye sockets, visualizing light entering your eyes. Then rub your face with your hands and use your palms to brush your hair from the top to the bottom. Now you should feel energized and ready to greet the day.

ENERGY THROUGH BREATH

Much of the time you take shallow breaths that penetrate only as far as the upper part of your lungs. By adapting the way you breathe so that you draw air deep down into your body, you can ensure that a rich supply of oxygen reaches your blood to energize and revitalize you. Breathing exercises that help you to alter your breathing pattern so you can use your lungs to their full capacity will provide an excellent preparation for the day ahead.

If you are someone who would prefer not to do physical exercises first thing in the morning, perhaps breathing exercises are the thing for you. If you take a little time to concentrate on your breathing at the beginning of each day, you'll feel more energized, alert, lucid and clear-headed. Once you get into the habit of breathing deeply – all the time, not just in the morning – you will find it helps to enhance your overall levels of energy and well-being. Breathing more deeply – and efficiently – also steadies the nervous system, massages the abdominal organs, which aids digestion and waste elimination, and reduces feelings of anxiety.

The following exercises, "complete yoga breath" and "lucidity breath" (on page 28), both encourage you to make more use of your diaphragm, the large sheet of muscle just under the lungs that separates the chest from the abdomen. Lucidity breath is also called *kapalabhati*, which can be translated as "skull shining". This graphically describes its ability to bring "mental lightness". The technique floods the body with oxygen and expels carbon dioxide and toxins from the lungs. It also stimulates the heart, which enhances circulation, and massages the internal organs. It is widely used by yoga practitioners as a *kriya*, or cleansing exercise, because it cleanses and purifies the air passages and the body's energy channels.

COMPLETE YOGA BREATH

Although the area within the lungs is one continuous space, for the purposes of this exercise it may help to imagine that each lung is divided into three separate compartments: lower, middle and upper. Complete yoga breath fills and empties each of these parts in turn. At the top of your inhalation, your lungs should feel completely full of air; at the bottom of your exhalation, your lungs should feel completely empty. Of course, in physiological terms, it is impossible to completely fill or totally empty the lungs, but most people find this visualization helpful. Your breath should flow evenly and steadily – don't be tempted to cram air into your lungs or force it out. Never strain. On your inhalation, imagine you are drawing in energy, vitality and light, which then permeates your entire being. On your exhalation, imagine your breath is carrying fatigue and impurities out of and away from your body. You can practise complete breathing lying on your back, but you may find it easier if you sit cross-legged on the floor.

Sit in a cross-legged position with your palms resting on your abdomen just below the navel. Take a few normal breaths, then inhale deeply through your nose, drawing air into the lower part of the lungs. Feel your abdomen balloon out beneath your hands. Move your hands up to rest on the area immediately below your ribs. Without pausing, continue your inhalation, drawing air into the middle part of your lungs. You should feel a small move-ment under your hands as your diaphragm moves down a little further. Cross your arms and place your fingertips immediately below your collarbones. Without pausing, continue your inhala-tion, drawing air into the upper part of your lungs. Feel your col-larbones rise slightly (but don't tense your shoulders).

Now that you have completed one entire inhalation, pause for a few moments and then exhale slowly and steadily from the upper, middle and lower parts of your lungs until you feel that you have expelled all the air. Repeat this inhalation and exhalation five times, aiming for a smooth and continuous flow of air.

Moving your hands from your abdomen to your ribs and then to your collarbones helps to guide you through the movements of complete breathing, but once you are familiar with the exercise, you can keep your hands resting on your knees.

"Imagine your breath dissolving into the all-pervading expanse of truth." Sogyal Rinpoche

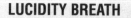

LUCIDITY BREATH

The following exercise is one of the most invigorating forms of breathing practised in yoga, guaranteed to bring lucidity and energize you in the morning. Unlike other yoga breathing techniques, it is fast and rhythmic, instead of slow and steady. The emphasis is on exhalation rather than inhalation. When you practise this for the first time, you should concentrate on your exhalations, which are forceful and pumping, and forget about your inhalations, which happen automatically.

When you have mastered this action, you can bring your awareness to the more subtle in-breath. If you are not used to the technique, the rapid breathing involved can make you dizzy or light-headed. If this happens, stop and breathe slowly and deeply through your nose. Avoid this exercise if you are pregnant, or suffer from cardiovascular problems, high blood pressure, depression, panic attacks, anxiety, epilepsy or diabetes, or have had recent abdominal surgery.

Sit in a cross-legged or other meditative posture (see pages 80–1). Take a couple of normal breaths, then inhale through your nose, drawing air deep down into your abdomen. Now exhale sharply through your nose – imagine that the force of the air is sufficient to blow out candles on a birthday cake. To do this you will need to contract your abdominal muscles. After doing so, your diaphragm will rise suddenly. You can feel this movement by placing your hand on your lower ribs.

Let your abdominal muscles relax briefly – as you do so air will be drawn into your lungs. Repeat the pumping exhalation followed by the automatic inhalation four times in rhythmic bursts. You should be able to hear the air coming through your nostrils. Four exhalations count as one round. Try to do a total of four rounds. Return to your normal way of breathing and spend a few moments enjoying the feeling of mental clarity and stillness. Now stretch your body before you stand up and get on with your day.

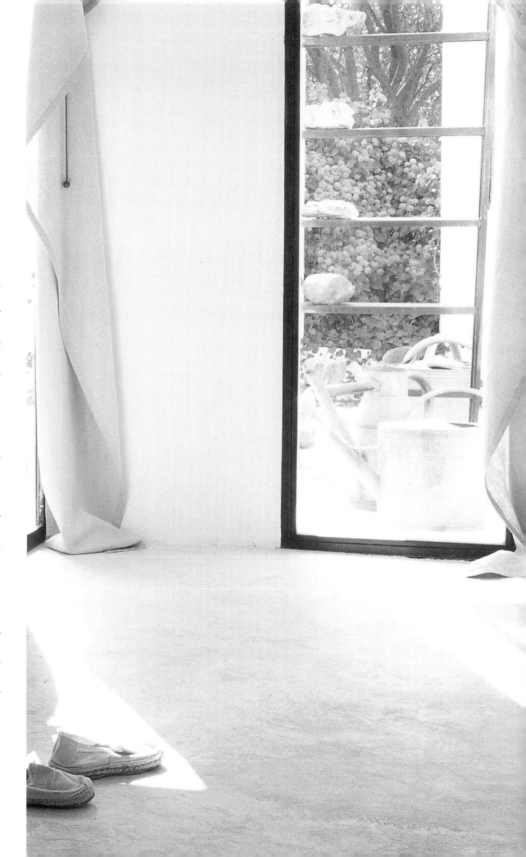

ESTABLISHING FOCUS

A wonderful way to achieve focus, energy and clarity for the day ahead is to start with a short meditation session. The following analogy, taken from Zen Buddhism (see page 64), helps to explain why meditation is beneficial: the mind is like the surface of a pool of water and our thoughts are like the wind. All the time the wind blows, the surface of the water is distorted by ripples. For the water to reflect clearly, like a mirror, the wind must stop blowing and the water must become still. Likewise, for the mind to exist in its true state, it must reach a point of perfect unbroken calm that is undisturbed by thought.

The best time to practise meditation is before you leave for work or, if staying at home, just prior to starting your daily tasks. If you practise it three or four mornings a week, you'll soon notice positive results such as a calmer outlook and increased concentration throughout the day. The following method, "breath counting", involves counting your breaths in cycles of 10. This gives instant feedback: as soon as your thoughts start to wander, you lose count of your breaths and so you can deliberately return your attention to counting. The breath counting technique may seem deceptively simple to people who are new to meditation. Many people find it difficult to concentrate even for short periods of time. You may be distracted by an itch, or a desire to move, or find that random thoughts or worries intrude. You may find that memories pop up during meditation. Whatever is going on in your mind, the aim is the same – to return your attention to breath counting. Don't worry if you lose count, simply start at one again.

HOW TO ESTABLISH FOCUS THROUGH MEDITATION

Find a peaceful space and sit in a comfortable meditation position (see page 80–1) or kneel astride a bolster. Rest your right hand in your left hand with palms facing up. Place the thumb tips lightly together to form an oval space between thumbs and fingers. With your hands in this position, hold them next to your lower abdomen, resting your arms lightly on your upper thighs. This position helps to turn your attention inward. Remain still with eyes lowered and gaze resting on the ground just in front of you. Breathe through your nose and count each exhalation only. Count up to 10 and then go back to one. Do this for 5–10 minutes at a time. When you finish, allow yourself a few moments to stretch, yawn and reorientate yourself before the day begins.

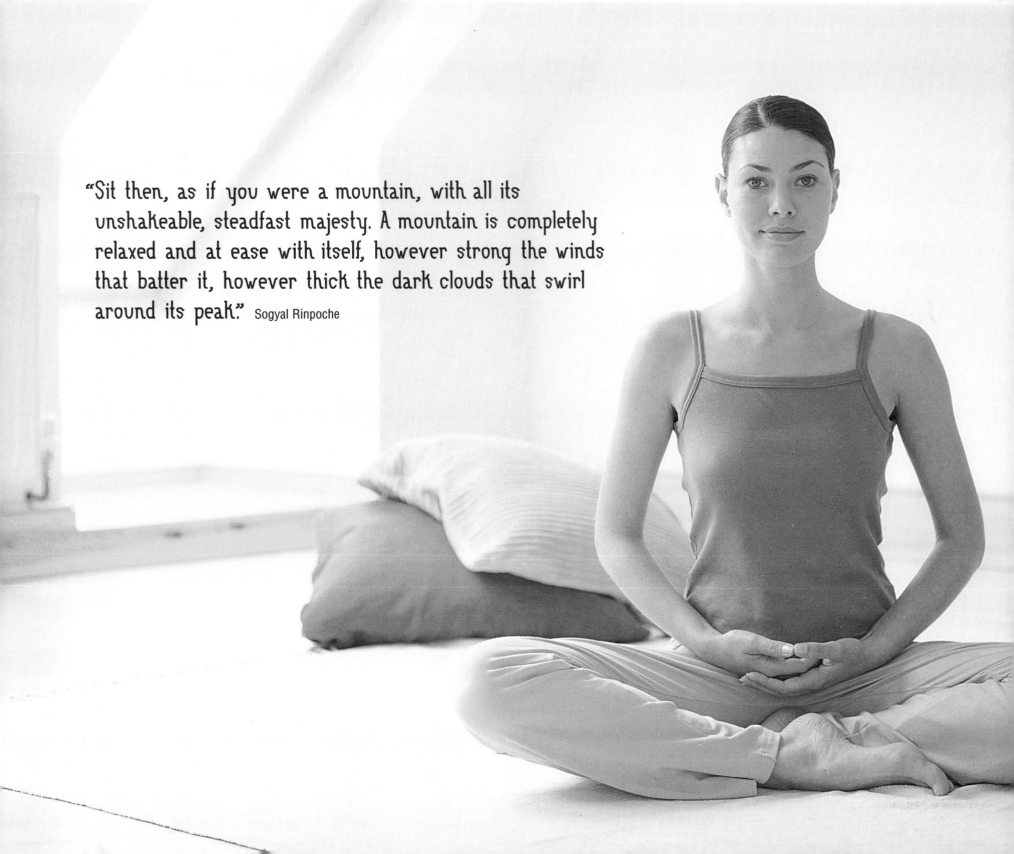

"Sit then, as if you were a mountain, with all its unshakeable, steadfast majesty. A mountain is completely relaxed and at ease with itself, however strong the winds that batter it, however thick the dark clouds that swirl around its peak." Sogyal Rinpoche

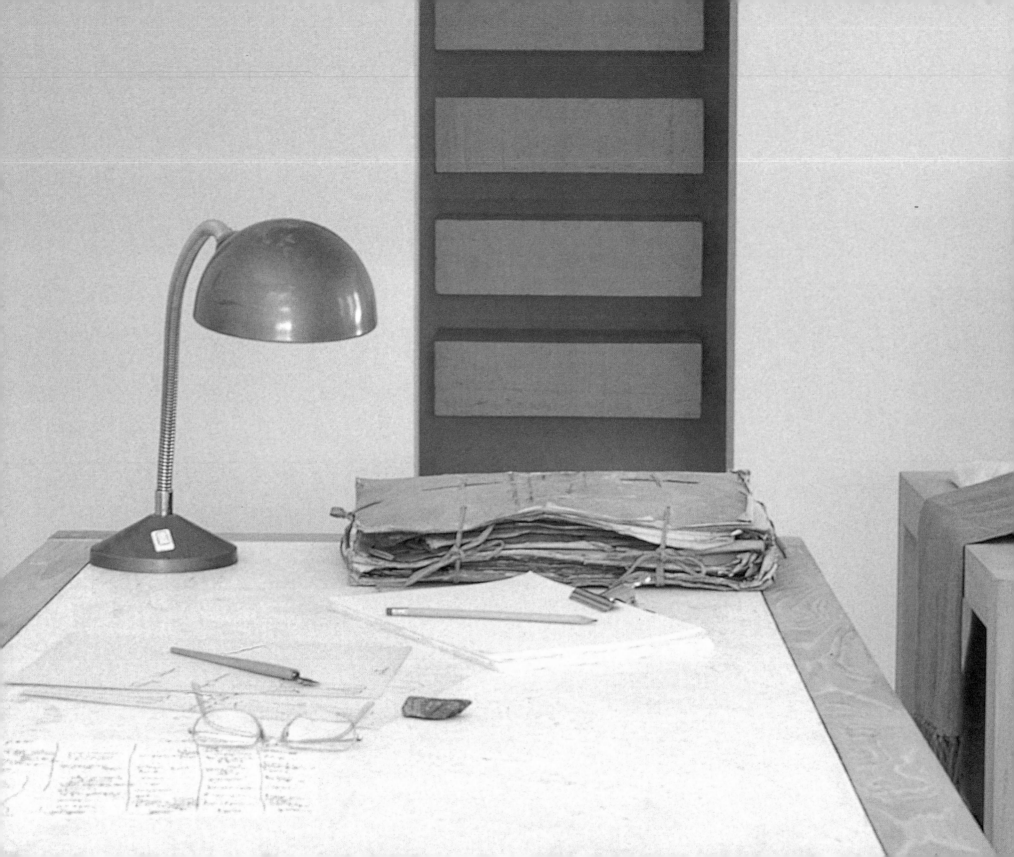

WORKING

Work can bring meaning and purpose to life and may even be a route to personal

and spiritual development; in Buddhism work or "right livelihood" is part of the

eightfold path to enlightenment. But the stress and rush of modern working life

can place huge obstacles along this path.

This chapter looks at ways to enhance your experience of work by overcoming

stress and its many side effects, and by managing your work through meditative

techniques that focus and discipline the mind. Methods derived from yoga, reiki

and acupressure can keep your body supple and feeling good throughout the day.

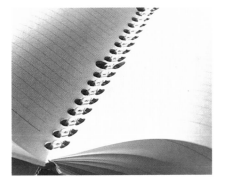

STAYING FOCUSED

The ability to maintain focus, to direct your attention unwaveringly to one thing for long periods, is one of the most useful skills for a successful working life. According to yoga teaching, if the body is nourished by free-flowing life-force energy (*prana*), a state of relaxed concentration comes naturally. The following sequence encourages the free flow of *prana* and aids concentration. The ideal time to do this sequence is in the morning before you leave for work, or during a break at work. But if this is not possible, it is also effective when practised in the evening.

The grounding posture (step 1) helps you to feel centred and rooted. The balancing posture (step 2) aids focus by forcing the mind to eliminate distractions. The inverted poses (steps 3 and 4) aid concentration by increasing blood flow to the brain. The first two steps are safe for everyone. But avoid the inverted poses if you suffer from high blood pressure, or ailments of the neck or head, or find the postures difficult or uncomfortable. Stay in each pose for as long as is comfortable. Come out of each pose slowly and gently. Breathe smoothly and deeply throughout. If you feel dizzy, short of breath or uncomfortable, come out of the posture and lie on your back, completely relaxed, for a few minutes.

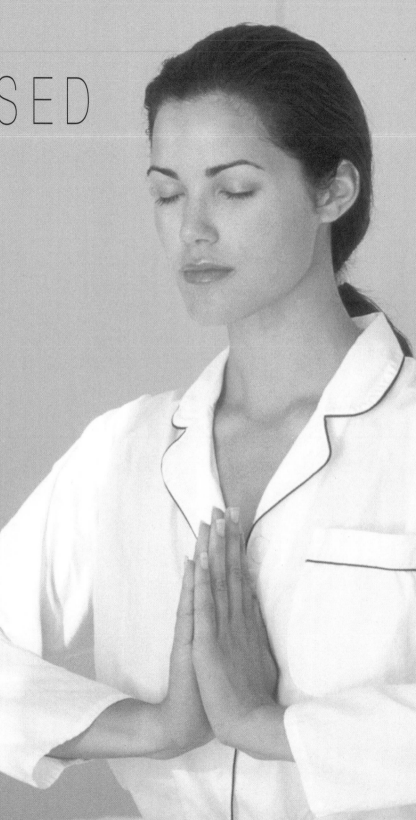

FOCUSING SEQUENCE

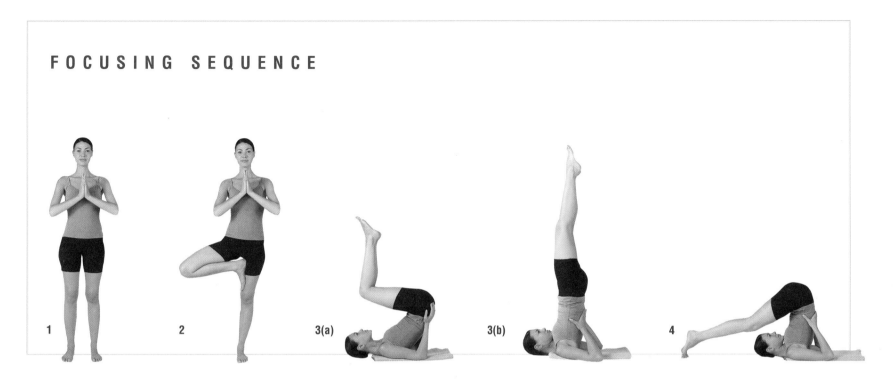

1   1   3(a)   3(b)   4

1 Stand with your feet parallel and close together and your arms by your sides. Keep your neck and shoulders relaxed and make sure your pelvis is neither tilting backward nor forward. Bring your palms together as if in prayer. Be completely steady and still. As you stand in this pose, close your eyes and imagine your feet growing roots into the ground.

2 Raise your right knee and turn out at 90 degrees. Gently place the sole of your right foot on the inside of your left leg as high as possible, while maintaining good balance. With palms in the prayer position, focus softly ahead. Repeat on the other side.

3 (a) Lie on your back on a folded blanket with your head on the floor and your shoulders on the blanket. Bring your knees to your chest and use your abdominal muscles to raise your legs and hips off the ground. Support your lower back with your hands. (b) Straighten your legs up to the ceiling and raise your body into a full shoulderstand. Support your weight on your shoulders, head and upper arms and continue to support your lower back with your hands.

4 Hinging at your hips, take your legs over your head and rest your toes gently on the floor behind you in the plough position. Keep supporting your lower back with your hands. Come down by gently uncurling your body until you are flat on your back.

MAINTAIN FOCUS

DISCIPLINE YOUR MIND

OVERCOME STRESS

"Flow around obstacles, don't confront them. Don't struggle to succeed. Wait for the right moment." Tao Te Ching

TRANQUIL WORKSPACES

Whether your workspace is a desk in an office building, or an area of the home set aside for work, writing, accounts, hobbies or study, you can apply the principles of feng shui, the Chinese art of object placement, to ensure that your working area fulfils basic criteria for comfort and efficiency. A fundamental principle of feng shui is that rooms must be free of clutter if positive energy (*chi*) is to flow freely. So the first step is to clear away untidy piles of books, boxes or files, and to ensure that aisles and doorways are kept unobstructed and that surfaces are not obscured by papers.

ADJUST YOUR WORKSTATION

Feng shui practitioners advise that we should observe how our mood and energy levels change as we enter our workspace. If it makes you feel stressed, depressed or alienated, simple adjustments to your workstation can make dramatic differences. For example, you could change the position of your desk or sit on the other side of the desk. Try to avoid having your back to a doorway, as this creates subconscious feelings of vulnerability. Choose a position with your back to a wall where you have a commanding view of the room or can see out of a window. If this is not possible, place a mirror on your desk to reflect the room, doorway or window behind you.

Safety and comfort are important considerations. A badly positioned chair and desk not only leads to poor posture, often resulting in neck and back ache and arm strain, but also restricts the body's internal flow of *chi*, causing fatigue and difficulty concentrating. Your chair should be stable, fully adjustable – to keep you in an aligned posture (see page 44) – and give good support to the lower spine. Ensure you have plenty of legroom and can rest your forearms flat on the desk with your shoulders relaxed.

PERSONALIZE YOUR SPACE

Place photographs, pictures or objects around the workspace that have personal significance for you. If you often feel stressed at work, place a restful or meditative image on your desk, such as a photograph of a picturesque landscape, lake or waterfall. Use this as a reminder to practise breathing (see pages 82–5) or visualization techniques when your day gets hectic. Natural objects enhance the flow of energy through a room. Choose a rock or crystal for your desk or place a beautiful plant or a vase of fresh

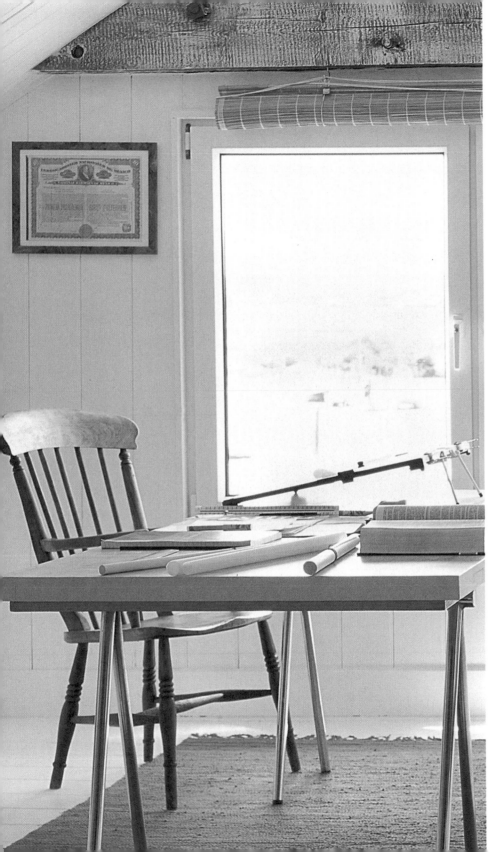

flowers near you (never keep dead or dying plants around you at work as they will depress energy in a room). Fountains represent continuous turnover and have a positive effect on productivity. If co-workers agree, introduce natural sounds and smells. Wind chimes placed in a doorway create beautiful and relaxing sounds. Essential oils, such as orange, lemon or tangerine, are uplifting. You can burn essential oils in an oil burner, or use an atomizer to spray essential oils mixed with water around the room.

USE COLOUR AND LIGHT

Consider changing the colour scheme in your workspace. Blue is soothing and tranquil, yellow is uplifting and aids communication, and red is stimulating and encourages action. If you cannot overhaul the design of your office, introduce colour in small ways to your immediate area. For example, use pictures, bright screen savers on your computer or a desk lamp with a coloured shade.

Lighting levels also have a significant effect on mood and energy flow. Don't rely on overhead fluorescent lighting as your sole source of light. Where possible, work in natural light or position a lamp to one side to provide additional illumination.

 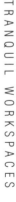

DISCIPLINE AT WORK

Discipline is a much maligned concept in the West. We associate it with rigid and restrictive rules and codes of behaviour that we automatically want to resist. The Buddhist idea of discipline is very different; it involves simplifying life to its core elements, thus enabling you to identify what is truly important. The following four techniques use Buddhist principles of discipline to help you to bring clarity to your working day.

UNDERSTAND YOUR PURPOSE

Consider the following story. Three men are working together on the same task when an observer asks each man what he is doing. The first man answers: "I am working." The second man answers: "I am laying bricks." The third man answers: "I am building a cathedral." The first two men have a limited view of their work. The third man not only sees an obvious point to his actions but also has a clear yardstick by which to measure his progress.

Taking an overview of the purpose of your work gives you a sense of positivity, direction and meaning, and helps you to organize yourself. Next time you start a new task, ask yourself: "How will this help me to complete my work?" If a task doesn't seem relevant, try to deprioritize or shed it altogether. For example, cut down on the telephone calls you make or the memos you write, and try to extricate yourself from office politics. Focus, instead, on the core tasks that can help you to achieve your goal. Never lose sight of the purpose of the job you are doing.

TREAT ALL TASKS AS EQUAL

Once you have streamlined your job by identifying its purpose, regard all your remaining tasks as equal. An important aspect of Buddhist practice is to consider everything of equal importance and merit. In the words of the Buddha: "What is little becomes much." At work, we regularly make value judgements without even being aware of them. Subconsciously, we divide our tasks into compartments: boring, interesting, difficult, easy, stressful and so on. Naturally, we then neglect the "negative" tasks and concentrate on the "positive" ones. As a result, periodically we are faced with a build-up of the tasks that we don't want to do.

It's well worth imagining how your working life could be transformed if your attitude to every aspect of your job was one of utter equanimity. How would it be if you could do your most hated tasks with complete absorption and concentration? This may seem difficult to achieve, but all it requires is the recognition that feelings of frustration, boredom or impatience arise from the way you habitually perceive a task – not the task itself.

Try this test. Choose a task that you normally dislike or put off. Now do it fully and completely, giving it your single-minded attention. Don't rush it or feel resentful. Find value in the task and remind yourself that it is just as important and deserving of your time as any other. When the task is complete, don't give yourself a reward or congratulate yourself on having got through something unpleasant. Simply accept that the task is done. The aim of this experiment is to hold your usual emotional responses in check and explore how it is possible to complete work in a dispassionate way. If you adopt this approach all the time, it will help you to work with less stress and more efficiency.

STEADY YOUR THOUGHTS

Another way to discipline yourself at work is to organize your mind. Yoga texts compare the mind to a cage full of excited monkeys. Even when you're busy doing one task, your thoughts may be leaping ahead to the next task, meeting or telephone call, or you might be analyzing how fast or well you're working, so that instead of being immersed in the task itself, you have a judgmental commentary running in your head. Alternatively, you may be preoccupied with something completely unrelated to work.

In the long term, the key to becoming more focused is to practise meditation (see page 78). In the short term, you can clear your mind by using a meditative technique known as "centring". This helps you to achieve steadiness and focus at any point in a busy day. First, spend a few moments deciding what you want to achieve from centring. Be as specific as possible. Do you want to feel more alert? Do you want to relax? Do you want to concentrate? Once you are clear about your aim, choose a word that fits what you want to achieve such as "alert", "relax" or "focus".

To practise centring, sit back in your chair and say the word "calm" as you inhale and say your chosen word as you exhale. You don't have to close your eyes or change your breathing. Focus or "centre" on the two words by repeating them in time with your breath for about a minute (no longer, as you need to train your mind to centre quickly). If you get distracted, just return your thoughts to the two words you are repeating. When a minute has passed, reflect on the exercise and see how it has worked. Ask yourself whether you feel any different – physically, mentally or emotionally. If you don't notice an improvement, don't worry. Keep practising it at different times (around five times a day). Eventually your mind will become trained and will respond more readily to centring practice. Make sure you always do all three stages: deciding what you want to achieve; centring itself; and reflecting upon the results.

DISENGAGE FROM DISTRACTIONS

A major problem in working life is that you are often expected to perform many different jobs at once. As the brain is poor at coping with multiple demands, this can be extremely stressful. One coping strategy is to list your tasks and perform them one by one. It also helps to train your mind to get rid of all unnecessary distractions. The following technique is specifically designed to help you to identify distractions and actively let them go. It takes around 15 minutes and can be practised before or after work, or in your lunch hour. Sit in a comfortable place and concentrate on

"Employment is nature's physician, and is essential to human happiness." Galen

the breath entering and leaving your nostrils. Don't change your breathing – just observe the sensation of air moving in and out. If you become distracted from the sensation of your breath, turn your attention to the distraction. It may be a sensation, such as an itchy leg; a thought, such as "what shall I have for lunch?"; or an emotion, such as irritation. Allow yourself to classify and name the distraction. For example: "My emotion is one of irritation with myself for not being able to concentrate." Now, firmly direct your thoughts back to the movement of breath within your nostrils. This takes a conscious effort of will and is known as active disengagement. If it helps, say the word "later" to whatever is distracting you. Now concentrate on your breath for the rest of the 15 minutes, using active disengagement whenever you need to.

By practising this technique every day, you quickly learn to be aware of what is going on in your mind (we are often oblivious to background mental chatter) and then to disengage yourself. This leaves you free to concentrate fully on another activity. It is also useful to ask yourself at intervals throughout the day: "What has my mind been doing for the last two minutes?" Actively identifying your mental activity helps you let go of it.

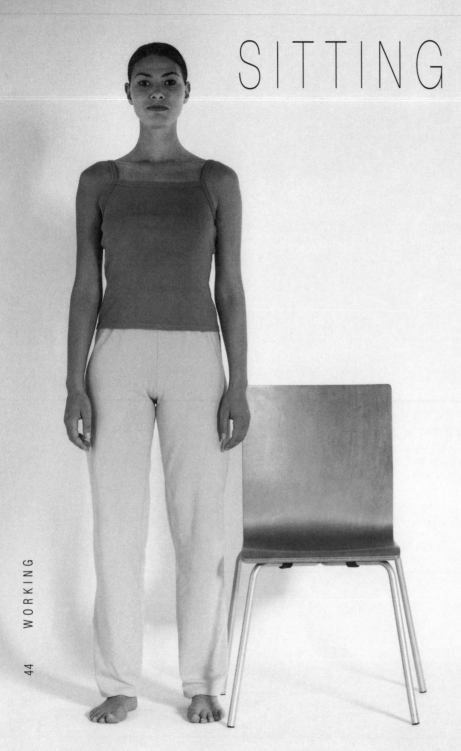

SITTING AND STANDING

The body is designed to move around rather than to sit still all day, so it's no surprise that those who habitually slump in a chair or stand badly develop back pain, postural problems, repetitive strain injury, and other health disorders. Yoga can help you to retrain your body to maintain a posture in which the muscles are relaxed and the body is aligned. This way you preserve your health and vitality and feel far less tired at the end of the day.

Postural flaws, such as slouching, cause muscle tension in the neck, shoulders and back because of the effort expended in supporting the head. It takes less effort if the head is aligned and rests on top of the spine. Postural changes can seem awkward at first, but if you persevere they'll soon start to feel more natural.

The following positions – "the mountain pose" and "the Egyptian pose" – are derived from yoga postures, and help you to maintain correct alignment of the body. To start, relax all muscles except those needed to hold you in a sitting or standing position. Feel the tension drop away from your shoulders, arms and legs.

THE MOUNTAIN POSE (Opposite)

Stand with your feet parallel and slightly apart. Spread your toes and be aware of the contact your feet make with the ground. Close your eyes and move your body in small circles until you find your natural centre, neither tipping backward nor forward. Aim to keep your head, neck, spine, pelvis, legs and feet in a straight line and weight distributed evenly over both feet. Keep your shoulders relaxed, chin level and head balanced easily on your neck.

THE EGYPTIAN POSE (Right)

Sit on a chair with your feet flat on the floor, feet and knees together or slightly apart. Keep your spine and neck in a straight line and your head perfectly balanced on top of your neck, rather than tipping forward or backward. Sit tall but without being rigid. Centre the weight of your upper body on your sitting bones rather than on the fleshy parts of your buttocks (to find your sitting bones, sit cross-legged on the floor and rock from side to side).

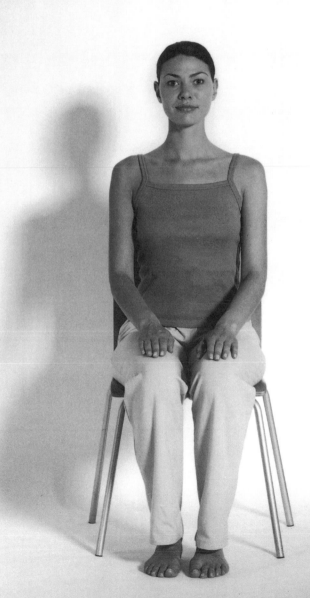

INSTANT CALM

One of the time-honoured methods of calming the mind is a yoga technique known as alternate nostril breathing. If, at any point during the working day, you are nervous, stressed, angry or feel that your thoughts are spiralling out of control, practise this simple exercise to restore your sense of perspective. The technique of alternate nostril breathing is straightforward and consists of inhaling through one nostril and exhaling through the other. To aid this process, use your fingers and thumb in a position known as *Vishnu mudra* to close each nostril in turn.

According to yogic theory, alternate nostril breathing brings balance to two energy channels (*nadis*) in the body. These *nadis*, *ida* and *pingala*, are opposite in character. *Ida nadi* is associated with your resting state. *Pingala nadi* is associated with your alert state. By breathing equally through left and right nostrils you balance the flow of energy (*prana*). This brings a state of harmony and equilibrium to the nervous system and dissipates anxiety.

Alternate nostril breathing may take a bit of practice before you feel comfortable doing it naturally. But just a few sessions at home can make the technique familiar enough to use to ease tension at work. The only prerequisite is that both nostrils are clear, so you may have to avoid alternate nostril breathing if you have a cold or hayfever and a blocked nose. Throughout the exercise, keep your breathing slow, deep, smooth and flowing. Take your breath right down into your abdomen (see page 26). Keep your facial muscles completely relaxed and concentrate your thoughts on the flow of your breath.

ALTERNATE NOSTRIL BREATHING

Sit upright in a straight-backed chair (see page 45) or cross-legged on the floor. Make the *Vishnu mudra* position with your right hand by folding your index and middle fingers into your palm. Rest your left hand on your left knee. Now close your right nostril with your right thumb and inhale deeply through your left nostril. Close the left nostril with the ring and little fingers. Hold your breath for a few moments. (Keep your thumb on the right nostril.) Release your thumb and exhale through the right nostril. Now inhale through the right nostril. Now close it with your thumb. Hold your breath for a few moments, then release your left nostril and exhale. This is one complete round of alternate nostril breathing. Aim to complete at least 10 rounds.

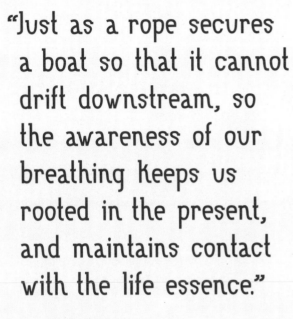

"Just as a rope secures
a boat so that it cannot
drift downstream, so
the awareness of our
breathing keeps us
rooted in the present,
and maintains contact
with the life essence."

The Bhagavad Gita

REIKI AT WORK

Reiki is a Japanese therapy that balances internal energy flow through the "laying on of hands". It is simple and safe to practise and is a great self-help technique that is particularly well suited to the workplace at times when you are suffering from stress, anxiety or headaches. *Rei* can be translated as "spiritual consciousness" and *ki* (like *chi* and *qi*) means "life-force energy".

As with many other Eastern therapies, reiki taps into this life-force energy, which is said to flow through and around all of us. When this energy becomes disrupted by negative thoughts and feelings, the cells and organs no longer function at their optimum level and you become prone to stress and illness. Reiki heals by causing blocked or negative energy to break up and dissolve.

FINDING YOUR TRUE SELF

Unlike therapies that involve movement, massage, pressure or manipulation, the success of reiki depends solely on the intent of the healer – whether a reiki master or yourself – and the healing presence of the hands on the body. Reiki is sometimes described as spiritual healing in that it puts you in tune with your true self. People who are trained in reiki receive an initiation process during which they are "reawakened" by a reiki master – from this moment onward they are able to transmit energy through their hands for the rest of their lives.

TREATING ENERGY IMBALANCES

Even if you haven't been initiated, you can still use reiki as a natural therapy by and on yourself. The following reiki hand positions are intended to treat energy imbalances in the head and throat. The first hand position (1) can ease headache, migraine, allergies, toothache and congestion in the upper respiratory tract. The second hand position (2) enhances mental functioning and eases headache, migraine and stress. The third hand position (3) stimulates energy and eases stress and nervousness. The fourth hand position (4) can ease headache, migraine and eye problems.

To practise reiki on yourself, first ensure that you are relaxed and sitting comfortably with your spine straight – you can stay sitting at your desk if you wish. Breathe through your nose and take your breath down into your abdomen. While practising reiki, concentrate on the place where you are resting your hands – energy is said to flow where the mind goes.

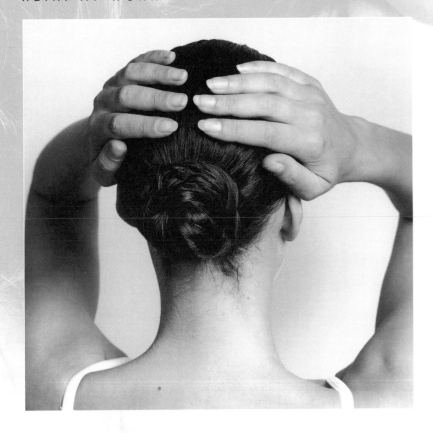
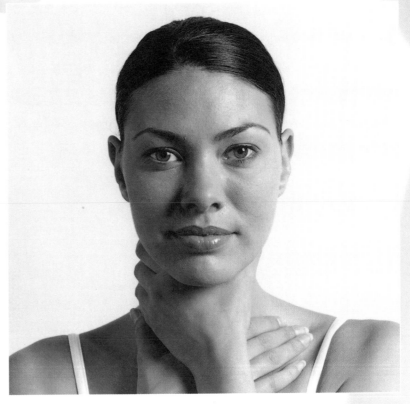

(1) Cover your face with your hands so that your fingertips are resting at the top of your forehead. (2) Bring your hands to your head with your fingertips resting at the midline of the crown and with your palms on either side of your head (above, left). (3) Place one hand gently around your throat and the other flat on your chest immediately below the first hand (above, right). (4) Bring your hands to the back of your head. Rest the heels of your hands at the base of your skull with your fingertips extending upward and bring the thumbs and fingertips of both hands together so that they form a rough triangle.

ACUPRESSURE RELIEF

Acupressure is an excellent self-help therapy that has been used for thousands of years to alleviate minor ailments. You can practise it while sitting at your desk to overcome some of the niggling problems experienced at work, such as eye strain, stiff shoulders and headaches. Acupressure, like acupuncture, is part of Chinese medicine. Symptoms of ill-health are attributed to blockages of life-force energy (*chi*) in the body. Both therapies seek to release blocked *chi* by acting on the 14 channels (meridians) that conduct *chi* around the body. But whereas acupuncture involves the use of fine needles, acupressure works by fingertip pressure.

There are acupressure points all over the body located at specific places on each meridian. Points are named after the meridian on which they lie. Most acupressure points are found in symmetrical pairs. Each point is used to treat a range of ailments. For example, for tired eyes, apply pressure to Liv 3 on the liver meridian. This point is on the top of the foot, two finger widths from the junction of the big and second toes. For lower back ache, apply pressure to Bl 23 or Bl 47, which lie on the bladder meridian on both sides of the spine at waist level. Bl 23 is two finger widths from the spine and Bl 47 is four finger widths from it.

HOW TO APPLY PRESSURE

When you practise acupressure, apply steady, firm pressure using the tip of the finger. Experts recommend a level of pressure that is halfway between pleasure and pain. Hold your finger (usually the middle one) at right angles to the surface of the skin and maintain pressure for around 20 seconds.

If you're not sure whether you are targeting the point accurately, probe the general area until you feel a sore, tender, numb or tingling sensation. This indicates that you've hit the right spot. Concentrate on directing the pressure to inside the part of the body that you are working on. Release the pressure for 10 seconds and then reapply for a further 20 seconds. Do this up to six times. Don't forget to press the point on each side of the body. Repeat this process several times over the next few hours or until your symptoms ease.

Make sure your nails are short, so you don't damage the skin, or use knuckle instead of fingertip pressure. (The eraser on the end of a pencil will also work!) If you are pregnant or suffering from a serious illness, always consult a practitioner of traditional Chinese medicine before using acupressure to treat yourself.

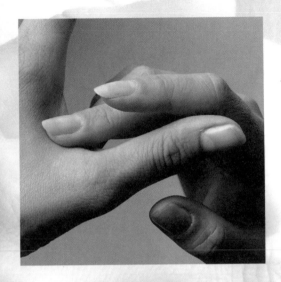

TENSION HEADACHE (Left)

To relieve a tension headache, press point LI 4. This is located on the large intestine meridian. LI 4 lies at the centre of the fleshy part between the thumb and the first finger on the top of your hand.

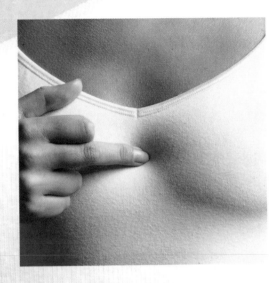

ANXIETY (Right)

If you are feeling anxious or upset, apply firm pressure to point CV 17 on the conception vessel meridian. This point is also known as the sea of tranquillity. It is located on the centre of the breastbone three thumb widths up from the base of the bone.

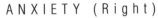

STRESS (Left)

As an antidote to stress, press point P 6 on the pericardium meridian. It lies between two tendons on the inner arm, two to three finger widths from the wrist crease. Clench your fist so it is easier to find the tendons.

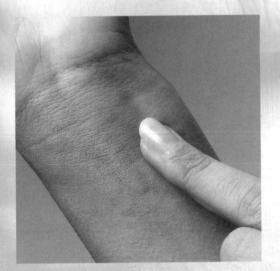

FATIGUE (Right)

To alleviate fatigue, press point St 36 on the stomach meridian, four finger widths below your kneecap toward the outside of your shinbone. Sp 6 on the spleen meridian is also useful – apply pressure three finger widths up from the anklebone, just off the edge of the shinbone.

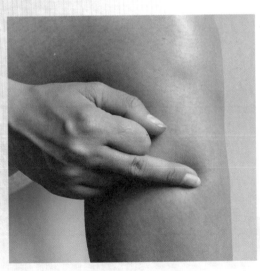

STAYING SUPPLE

Sitting at a desk all day can cause the body to lose its natural suppleness. Even simple actions such as bending over to touch your toes or sitting on the floor with a straight spine can become difficult. The best way to prevent these problems is to break up the working day with intervals of activity, such as walking around the block. The following sequence of stretches can also help. They need little space and can all be performed standing up. If you're pushed for time, you can modify the sequence to perform it sitting down (simply omit steps 5 and 6), as long as you remember to stand up and move about regularly.

The first stretch frees tension and encourages mobility in the shoulders, areas of the body that you may unconsciously tense or hunch while you work. The next four arm stretches improve posture and balance and give the shoulders, arms, wrists and fingers a quick work-out – ideal if you've been working at a keyboard for a long period. The forward bend loosens the neck, shoulders and back as well as improving blood flow to the brain. The last two positions improve circulation and suppleness in the legs and feet, helping to prevent blood pooling in the lower extremities when you sit for long periods. Do this sequence whenever you can.

SUPPLENESS SEQUENCE

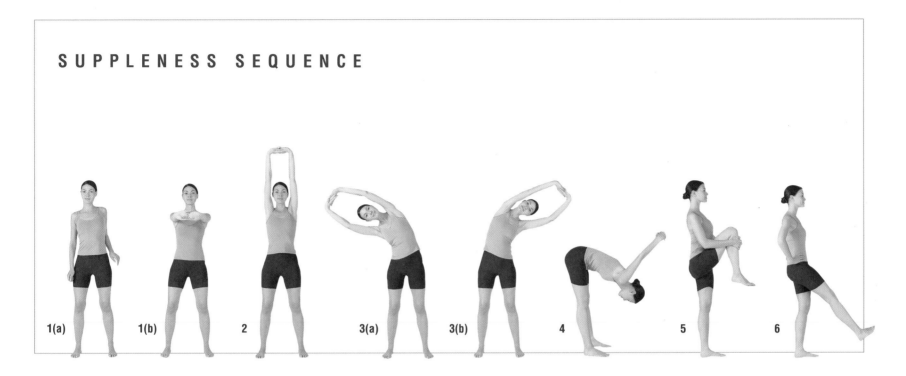

1(a) 1(b) 2 3(a) 3(b) 4 5 6

1 (a) Stand with your arms by your sides, feet a little way apart. Slowly rotate your shoulders in circles, first forward and then backward, at least five times. (b) Stretch your arms out in front of you and link your fingers. Push your palms out and away from you.

2 Lift your arms over your head. Stretch your body upward with your palms facing the ceiling. Keep your shoulders relaxed.

3 (a) Leading with the arms, stretch your upper body to the right. Return to step 2. (b) Repeat on the left. Lower your arms to your sides.

4 With feet hip-width apart, link your fingers together behind you and fold forward at the hips as far as you can. Keep your legs straight or slightly bent. Slowly bring your arms back and up. Stay like this for a few breaths and then return to a standing position.

5 Raise the right knee toward your chest. Clasp your hands just below the knee and hug your leg toward you. Repeat with your left leg.

6 Shift your weight on to your left leg and extend your right leg in a straight line in front of you. Circle your ankle three times clockwise and three times anticlockwise. Bring your right leg to the ground and repeat with your left leg.

IMPROVE POSTURE

INCREASE SUPPLENESS

FREE ALL TENSION

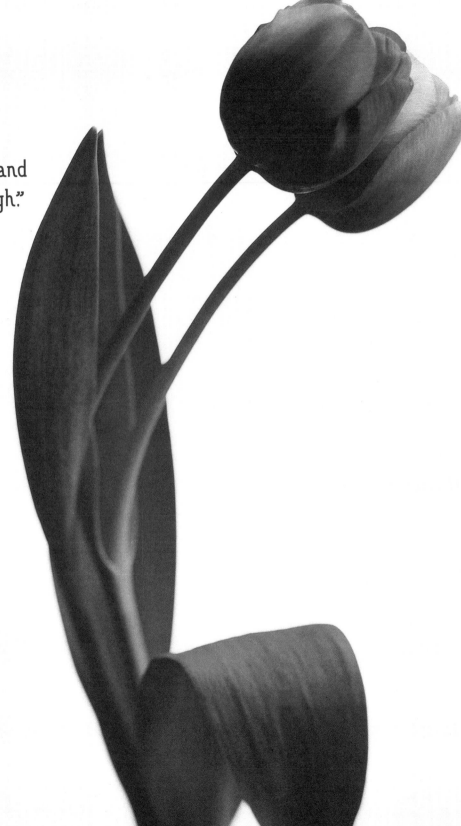

"Appreciate what you have and you will always have enough."

Tao Te Ching

STRETCH AWAY TENSION

Tension in the body while you are at work can be caused by a combination of mental and physical factors. For example, the stress of coping with a heavy workload and tight deadlines can cause tension and aching in the neck and shoulders. Poor posture, or sitting or standing in the same position for long periods, can lead to chronic stiffness and back pain. If your workstation is poorly designed it can force your body into a misaligned position and make you vulnerable to repetitive strain injury.

A good way to beat tension and stiffness at work is to do stretches that focus on key areas of the body. Most people, but particularly keyboard users, suffer from tension in three main areas: back, neck and shoulders. This can manifest itself in a variety of ways from a localized tingling sensation in one shoulder to general muscle stiffness, chronic headaches or backache.

Many of the following exercises concentrate on relieving tension in the long muscles of the neck and back using a combination of stretches and twists. You may also harbour tension around the jaw and eyes. The jaw joint (temporomandibular joint) is surrounded by muscles that enable a wide range of movements. If you sit with your jaws habitually clamped shut or you grind your teeth, these muscles can become chronically tense and give rise to facial pain and tension headaches. (Bear in mind that the only time the teeth need to meet is when we are chewing food.)

Start by identifying your personal tension spots. If, for example, you know that your neck is prone to stiffness or soreness, make the effort to practise some head rotations whenever you think about it or, if you want to be more disciplined, every hour on the hour. The important thing is to prevent discomfort occurring in the first place – not to wait until you are already in pain.

Most of the following exercises can be done sitting down. They only take a minute or two to perform. For a thorough stretch you can do them one after the other, if you wish. Otherwise, do them individually to relieve aches or pick those that target your tension hotspots and do them regularly. Most of the exercises are based on ancient yoga techniques – some thousands of years old.

TO RELIEVE NECK, BACK, ARM AND SHOULDER TENSION

The following back and arm stretch is fantastic if you have been sitting at a desk for a long time. Don't be embarrassed what your co-workers think – get them to join in too! Stand facing a chair

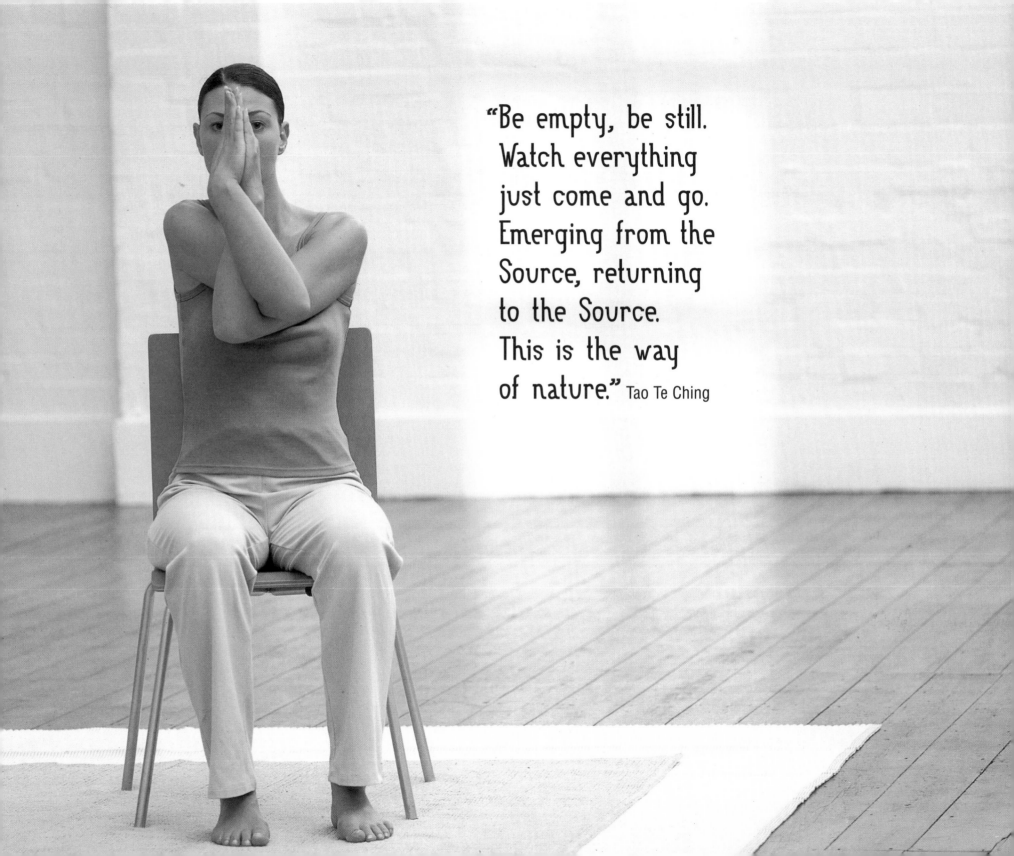

"Be empty, be still.
Watch everything
just come and go.
Emerging from the
Source, returning
to the Source.
This is the way
of nature." Tao Te Ching

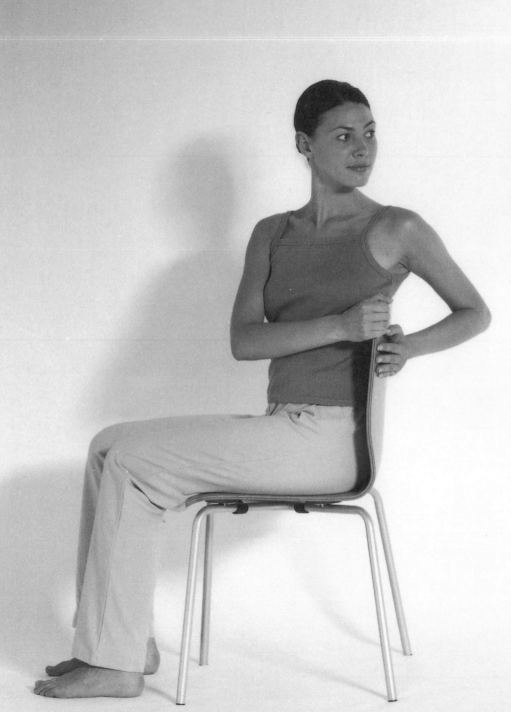

(ideally one that doesn't move – otherwise, just be careful!). Stretch your arms over your head and fold gently forward from the hips until your upper body is at right angles to your legs. Keep your knees slightly bent. Hold on to the back of the chair and make your neck and spine as long as possible. Stretch your fingers too (especially if you have been working at a keyboard). Hold the stretch for about 10 seconds.

To stretch your neck, sit on a chair and face the front, making sure your head is perfectly aligned with your neck and spine. Exhale and slowly turn your head as far to the right as possible without straining. Inhale and return to the centre. Exhale and slowly turn your head to the left. Repeat for up to 2 minutes.

To stretch your upper back, sit on a chair and drop your chin forward on to your chest, link your fingers and rest them on the back of your head (not your neck, though). Gently allow your arms to relax so that their weight stretches the muscles in your neck and back. Now turn your head to the right slightly and then to the left slightly. Come back to centre and release your hands.

If your arms and shoulders are feeling stiff, sit in a chair and cross your right arm over your left, palms facing up. Now bend your arms and twist your hands around so that you can rest part of your palms together. Direct your breath into the area between your shoulder-blades. To increase the stretch, lift your elbows higher. Repeat, crossing your arms the other way (see page 57).

TO RELIEVE BACKACHE

This is a simple but effective way to relieve backache caused by sitting hunched at a desk. Sit on a chair and slowly twist from your hips so your chest comes to face the back of the chair. Grasp either side of the chair back with your hands. Keeping your trunk straight, twist as far round as you can, and look over the shoulder that leads the twist. Repeat in the other direction (opposite).

TO RELIEVE EYE STRAIN AND FACIAL TENSION

Poor lighting, or staring at one object for hours on end without changing your depth of focus can lead to eye strain. If you have been staring at a computer screen, or reading reports all morning, the following exercises can ease eye strain. Look upward as if a clock hand is pointing to 12 o'clock just above eye level. Now look at 1 o'clock, 2 o'clock, 3 o'clock and so on until you have completed the full circle. (There should be no wrinkles in the skin at the back of the neck when you look up.) Repeat anticlockwise. Now rub your palms together vigorously and then cup them over your closed eyes so that all light is shut out. Rest your elbows on your desk or knees and tip your head forward. Breathe deeply.

The muscles of the face and jaw are prone to tension, too, especially if you habitually grind your teeth. The following exercise may help. Sit with your arms straight, spine tall and palms resting on your knees. As you inhale, bend forward slightly, open your mouth wide and stick your tongue out and down as far as you can. Open your eyes wide and gaze at the tip of your nose. Stretch your fingers and arms. Exhale forcefully, making the sound "haaa". Return to the start position. Repeat several times.

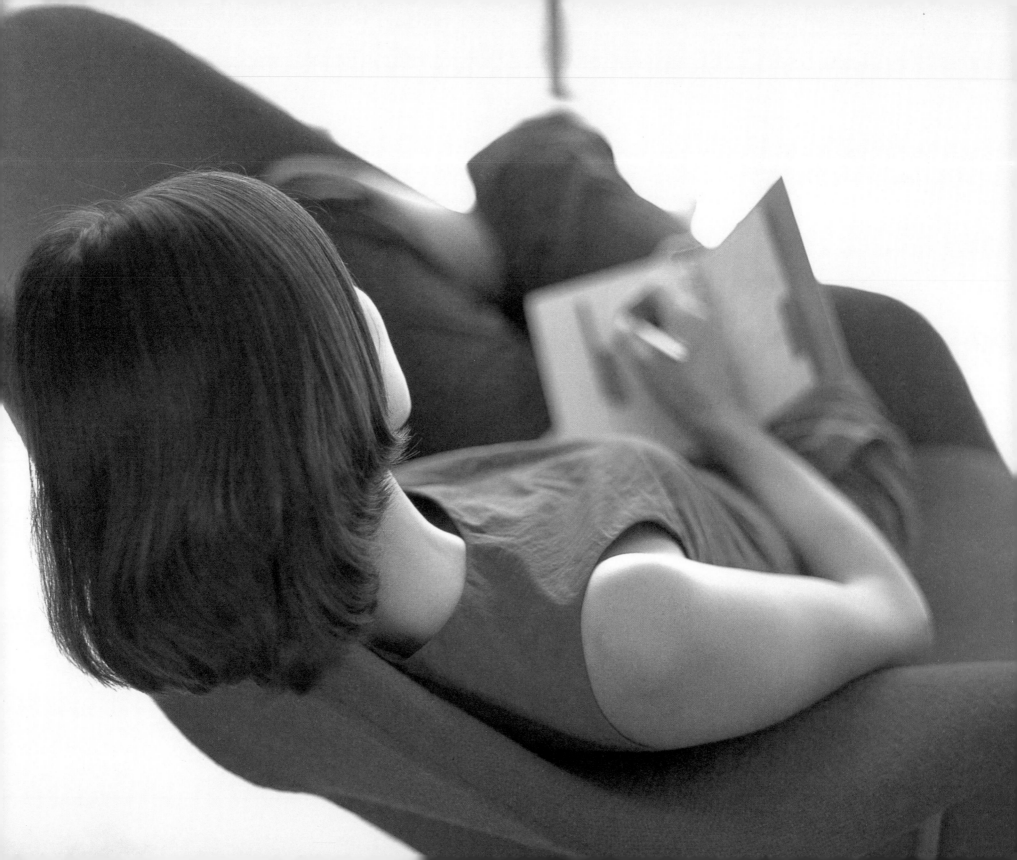

RELAXING

In today's hectic world of mobile telephones, fax machines and jam-packed work schedules, the art of relaxation is something that many of us have forgotten. True relaxation not only means resting the body, but also cutting yourself off, losing track of time, being absorbed in the moment and forgetting yourself completely.

This chapter explores the various ways in which you can do this, for example, through creative activities, spending time outside in a natural environment or rediscovering your childhood sense of fun and play. Eastern therapies such as qigong, yoga breathing and meditation are also explored as ways to bring the body and mind into harmony and ensure the greater relaxation of both.

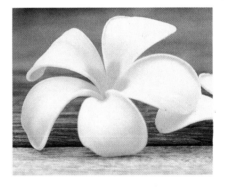

LETTING GO OF TIME

You don't have to be a slave to time *all* the time. The first step toward releasing yourself from the pressure of time and truly learning to relax is to be aware of the insidious effect that the clock can have on your sense of well-being. The relentless march of time often seems an inescapable factor of modern life. Even if you don't wear a wristwatch you are constantly being reminded of the hour by your alarm clock, radio and television. Common laments today are that "there aren't enough hours in the day" and that time is "short", "running out" or "against us".

To make matters worse, we go to bed at a predetermined hour, get up at a certain time (whether or not we feel rested) and clock in and out of work. Some companies now ask employees to account for increasingly small units of time, such as half and quarter hours, on timesheets. This puts pressure on people to be busy almost every minute of the day.

Yet the consequences of constantly racing against the clock can be punitive – anxiety, depression, high blood pressure and many other stress-related illnesses. To escape the tyranny of time, you need to change the way you think about it. Rather than being something immutable, with each second, minute and hour following inexorably, one after another, think of time as a purely social construct that you can alter to suit your own needs.

CREATE YOUR OWN CLOCK

It may help you to break free from the constraints of the clock if you understand how other cultures measure time. In some parts of India, time is described simply in terms of events or activities. For example, the time at which cowherds return home is known as "cattle-dust time". Some native North American languages contain no specific word for time, and no concept of second, minute or hour. Instead, there are words for moon, day and night, and sunset and sunrise. In the Andaman forests of India, people work to a "scent calendar", using the changing smells of plants and trees to indicate the passing months.

TAKE TIME OFF

Whenever you can, take time off from time. Leave your watch off and avoid asking others for the time. Instead, follow your own personal body clock. Eat when you are hungry, go to bed when you feel tired and sleep until you are rested. A good time to do this is when you're on holiday and can obey your internal clock for several days at a stretch. Many of us find it difficult to relax, even when taking a break from work – so resist the urge to give structure to your day with activities and outings. Give yourself the space to do nothing except watch time pass you by.

MANAGE YOUR TIME

Holidays aside, it's also important to claw back some time for yourself during the rest of the year. Teachers of Eastern disciplines such as yoga recommend meditation (see page 78) as a way of creating a "time-free" zone in your day. Western experts in time management suggest that you deliberately allocate time for exercise and leisure in your daily or weekly schedule – and try not to forego these sessions for any reason.

Another way to manage time is to create lists of achievable goals and prioritize them. Accept that you may not achieve them all and may have to strike off or delegate tasks that are lower down the list. Learn that it's normal to have a backlog of jobs to do and, finally, try to praise yourself for the tasks that you accomplish rather than criticize yourself for those that you don't.

THE ART OF ZEN

In the quest for mental and spiritual peace it may be helpful to alter the way you view the world and your place within it. One approach is through Zen, a form of Buddhism that originated in ancient China and spread to Japan. Zen is best thought of as a spiritual path or "way of being". The Zen idea of "self" differs from the Western concept. In the West, we see ourselves as individuals separate from (and often superior to) other people and the natural world. We define ourselves by our thoughts, feelings, relationships and jobs and believe we have a unique identity that we call "I". Zen Buddhists say this "I" is illusory. It is simply the ego, a false sense of self that prevents us from discovering our true nature. Zen aims to transcend the ego.

In Zen there is no distinction between you and the rest of the universe and no difference between you and your experiences. In many ways, this state of consciousness resembles that of babyhood in which life is experienced as a flow of pure awareness. According to a Zen saying: "No-one sees anything and no-one experiences anything — there is simply seeing and experiencing." We are our experiences. This idea of letting go of the ego is profoundly liberating — the only true way of achieving peace. As long as you identify yourself by your ego, you are in a trap in which you must dominate the world or suffer at its hands. You can lessen the grip of the ego by acknowledging that you form part of the universal flow of life and by practising *wu wei*.

This Zen concept means acting in accord with things as they exist — accepting the flow of life. An analogy would be trying to open a lock with a key that won't seem to turn. Rather than use force, we should adjust the key carefully until it slots into its proper place in the lock and turns naturally. Practising *wu wei* means going with the current rather than trying to swim upstream. This doesn't mean doing nothing, it means accepting life without desire, greed, longing, fear, criticism, resentment or judgment.

ZEN WALKING

Zen monks practise a discipline known as *kinhin*, Zen walking. This appears easy — you simply focus on the fact that you are travelling on foot. Yet it is also very difficult as your awareness of walking must exclude all other thoughts and sensations. In effect, *kinhin* is a moving meditation exercise that restricts your consciousness to a moment at a time, and it is profoundly relaxing.

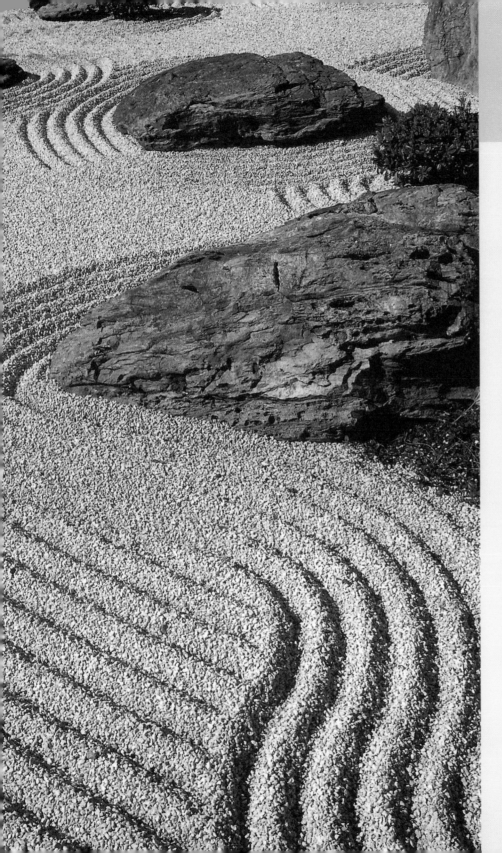

Plan a route that takes about 30 minutes at a fairly slow walking pace. Ideally, choose a quiet path that you know well – this helps to eliminate distractions such as the sound of traffic and wondering which way to go next. As you begin your walking meditation, note the sensation of your feet inside your shoes and feel the way your feet lift off and impact upon the ground. Identify the precise moment when each action begins. Slow your walk and bring your whole attention to the tiny movements your feet make as you lift, swing and lower them. Mentally repeat the word "left" as your left foot hits the ground and "right" as your right foot hits the ground. Focus softly at about three paces in front of you. Keep up this level of awareness for the duration of your walk.

It takes a little practice to achieve "mindfulness" – the Buddhist concept of being immersed in the moment. Signs that you are becoming mindful during *kinhin* are a sense that time is slowing down, allowing you to observe in an unhurried way the minutiae of each tiny foot action, and a feeling that your feet are dissolving, becoming lighter, or disappearing and reappearing. If you experience sensations like these don't be seduced or unnerved by them – simply return your attention to your walking.

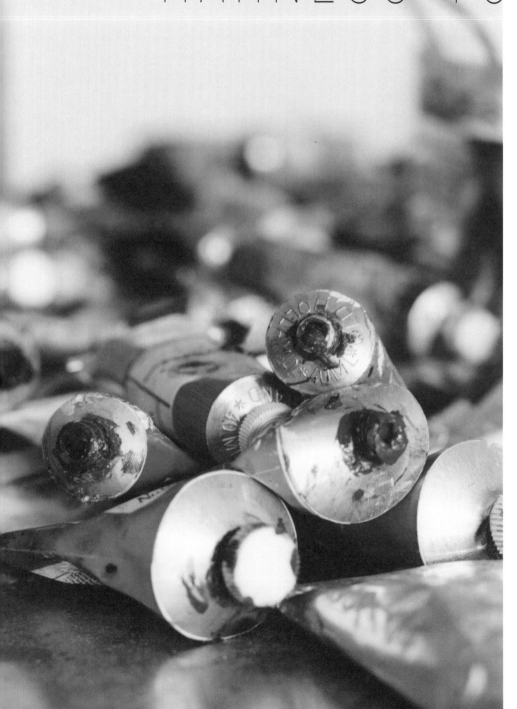

HARNESS YOUR CREATIVITY

Creativity is a way of expressing your higher self – that which Buddhists call your "Buddha-nature". Unlike many of your day-to-day activities creativity is not goal-orientated, it is not necessary for your physical survival and it is not something that is expected of you by others. Rather, it is something you do purely for the joy of self-expression. Imagine a potter at a wheel or a young child at play – both are totally absorbed in their tasks. This sense of being lost in the moment is good for you. It lifts you out of mechanical and habitual behaviour in which your mind is only half engaged and plunges you into a sense of "nowness".

BE AT EASE WITH YOUR CREATIVE SIDE

Although "nowness" is a Buddhist concept, it has been adopted by Western psychologists who refer to it as "the flow". People who have "flow" experiences are less aware of time (hours stream past as though they are minutes), they feel relaxed and at ease, free from feelings of self-consciousness and are totally in tune with themselves. Achieving "creative flow" is something that everyone can cultivate. But it's sometimes necessary to get rid of the following psychological obstacles first.

You may believe (albeit unconsciously) that you should only express yourself creatively if you can do it well. Perhaps you feel there is no point in writing a story unless it is good enough to be published, or that it is a waste of time painting a picture unless it is worthy of display. You may have internalized these beliefs during childhood, perhaps because of comments made by parents or school teachers. These beliefs can be powerfully inhibiting in adulthood as they can restrict your creative side.

FEEL FREE TO FAIL

To overcome this fear of failure, give yourself the freedom to be bad at something. Tell yourself that you will paint a picture or embroider a tapestry simply for the sake of artistic expression. It doesn't really matter what the end result will be like – the important thing is the process. Try to let go of your ego.

Another creative straitjacket is the preconception that artistic expression has a limited number of forms. Painting, literature or music may be the first subjects that spring to mind. However, creativity is wider than this. You can be creative by dancing, cooking a meal, taking a photograph, decorating a room, planting a flower-bed or telling a story. You also express yourself creatively in the way you work, make love or parent your children.

HOW TO GET STARTED

Getting started is often the most difficult aspect of creative work. It's easy to plan something but less easy to set that plan in motion. You may well feel that you have "more important" things to do. Unfortunately, these are most likely to be job-related or domestic tasks that do not bring you the same rewards as creative pursuits. Challenge your in-built mind set and consciously bring yourself to value the time you spend in creative pursuits as much as, if not more than, work or chores.

Resolve to spend a short amount of time pursuing a creative goal today. If you feel short of inspiration, try meditating, practising yoga, looking at a beautiful picture or listening to a stimulating piece of music. Alternatively, you may find that keeping a diary or journal is a good way to explore and generate creative ideas. Remember, you don't have to start out with a clear creative goal – just begin writing, doodling, dancing, painting or playing a guitar and see what happens.

HAVING FUN

It's easy to forget that life is also about having fun. If you're not careful, your days can be filled with tasks you feel compelled to complete, allowing simple enjoyment to fall by the wayside. You may tell yourself you don't have time for fun, that it won't pay the bills, clean the house or help you in your career. In other words, that fun is pointless. This approach can make life seem sterile. Eastern spiritual disciplines, such as Buddhism, emphasize "being" rather than "doing" – and having fun is one of the best ways of "being" there is. Pure fun and enjoyment are similar in many ways to the state of flow that people experience when they create music or meditate.

MAKE LEISURE TIME FUN TIME

In the quest to have fun, it's important to realize that even though you may assiduously dedicate time to leisure, this isn't necessarily the same as having fun. People often make the mistake of filling their leisure time with activities that have a clear goal. Examples include working out at the gym to lose weight and get fit; painting the spare room to increase the value of the home; or learning a new skill to enhance job prospects. These may well be beneficial, but they won't necessarily bring exhilaration and a sense of being immersed in the moment – oblivious to the passing of time. A simple test is: if you're motivated more by the end-result than by the process, you're probably not having fun.

LEARN TO LAUGH

Laughter has a positive effect on brain chemistry and mood, it relieves stress and tension and it unites the people around you. Resolve to keep smiling and laughing. Try to see the humour in every situation and laugh at it. If events seem to be conspiring against you, laugh at your bad luck instead of becoming bitter and resentful. Point out the humour of a situation to others.

If life seems joyless, try to understand why. One of the commonest reasons why many people don't have fun is that they feel self-conscious and are afraid of looking silly or of embarrassing themselves. If this applies to you, start by letting go of your inhibitions one by one. You don't have to behave completely out of character, just start pushing out your personal boundaries. For example, if you never tease people, crack jokes or tell amusing anecdotes for fear of looking foolish, start today.

HAVE A SECOND CHILDHOOD

Children are the experts at having fun. Compare a child's average day with that of an adult. Children devote much of their time to play, experimenting, being silly and simply enjoying themselves. Adults, on the other hand, are more likely to go through the day in a state of stressed momentum, weighed down by their responsibilities and worrying about unfinished tasks. Take a lesson from children and incorporate play into your daily life. Learn to do things that feel good, funny or exciting.

Every day, do something just for fun. It can be something as simple as smiling at a stranger, or stopping at a nearby park to have a go on the swings, feeding the ducks or throwing pebbles into a pond. Release yourself from goal-oriented activities and remind yourself that you don't always need a purpose.

Try running downhill at high speed, jumping into the deep end of a swimming pool, exploring a maze, drawing a silly picture or writing a comic rhyme. Include other people in your fun: play party games with friends, set up harmless practical jokes or have a water fight. If you need inspiration, spend some time with young children – and take your cues from them.

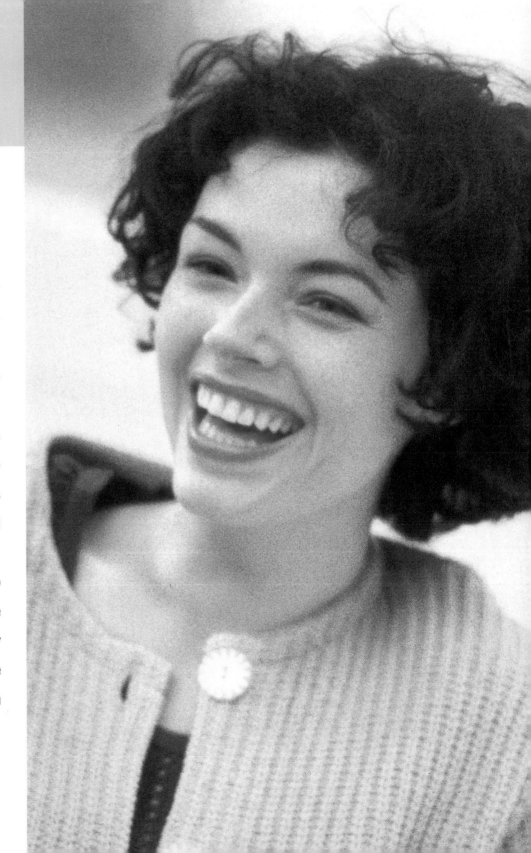

THIS SEQUENCE OF QIGONG MOVEMENTS IS A GENTLE WAY OF RELAXING THE MIND AND BODY AND ENHANCING YOUR AWARENESS OF YOUR INTERNAL FLOW OF ENERGY.

DAILY YOGA PRACTICE WILL HARMONIZE YOUR MIND, BODY AND SPIRIT, AND HELP TO ENGENDER A FEELING OF CONTENTMENT AND TOTAL WELL-BEING.

RELAXING QIGONG SEQUENCE

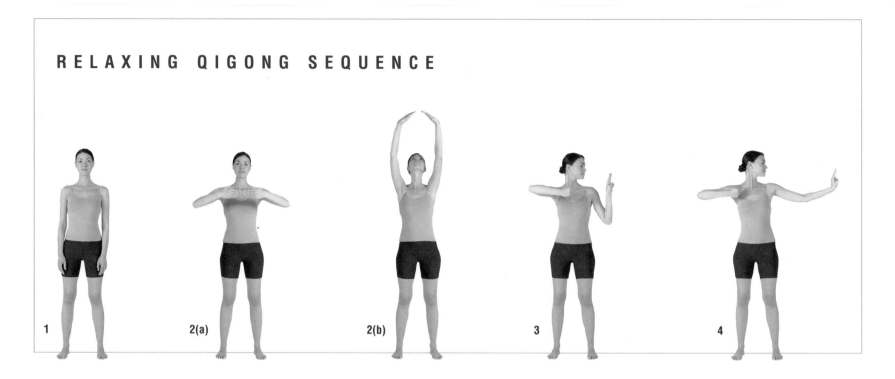

1   Stand with your feet shoulder-width apart and parallel or slightly turned out. Keep your knees slightly bent, your shoulders relaxed and your arms loosely by your sides. Imagine that your head is being drawn upward, that your feet are rooting downward and the middle part of your body is floating. This is the *Wu Chi* position.

2   (a) Exhale and stretch both arms out in front of you at shoulder height. Bend your elbows, palms facing inward, fingertips nearly touching. (b) Slowly raise your arms over your head, turning your palms to face out as they pass your face. Press your palms toward the ceiling and straighten your arms. Look up at your hands. Inhale and lower your arms. Repeat steps 2(a) and 2(b) eight times.

3   Stand in the *Wu Chi* position. Bend your elbows and raise your hands to chest height. Turn your left palm to face left and curl your thumb and ring and little fingers into your palm, leaving your index and middle fingers pointing straight up. Look to your left. Raise your right elbow at right angles to your body as if you are holding the bow of a bow and arrow. Curl your right fingers into your palm.

4   Exhale and extend your right elbow and your left arm as far to each side as possible, as if you are drawing a bow. Inhale and return your arms to the front of your chest. Repeat this on the other side. Do four movements on each side.

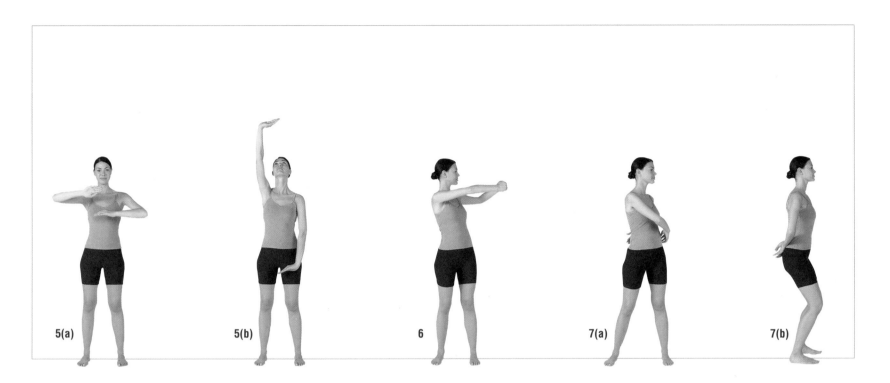

5(a)   5(b)   6   7(a)   7(b)

5 (a) Stand in the *Wu Chi* position. Bend your elbows and raise your hands to chest height. Rotate your right arm so that your palm faces out and your fingers point left. Rotate your left arm so that your palm faces down and your fingers point right. (b) Exhale and push your right palm up to the ceiling and your left palm down to the ground. Keep your arms straight and look up at your right hand. Inhale and bring your arms back to your chest. Repeat the movement on the other side. Do four movements on each side.

6 Stand in the *Wu Chi* position. Raise your arms in front of you to create a rough circle at chest height. Your palms face in and your fingertips are touching. Exhaling, swivel from your hips to face the left and bring your palms level with your face. Inhale and return to face the front, lowering your hands to chest height. Repeat the twist to the right. Do four movements on each side.

7 (a) Stand in the *Wu Chi* position. Swing your arms as you gently swing your body from left to right. As you swing to the left, tap your right kidney with the back of your left hand and tap the left side of your abdomen with your right palm. Do this four times on each side. (b) Stand in the *Wu Chi* position. Bend your knees slightly. Rest the backs of your hands in the small of your back over your kidneys. Bend your knees more and straighten them again letting your hands massage you as you move up and down. Do this eight times.

LET GO OF TIME

LIVE FOR THE MOMENT

LAUGH AND PLAY

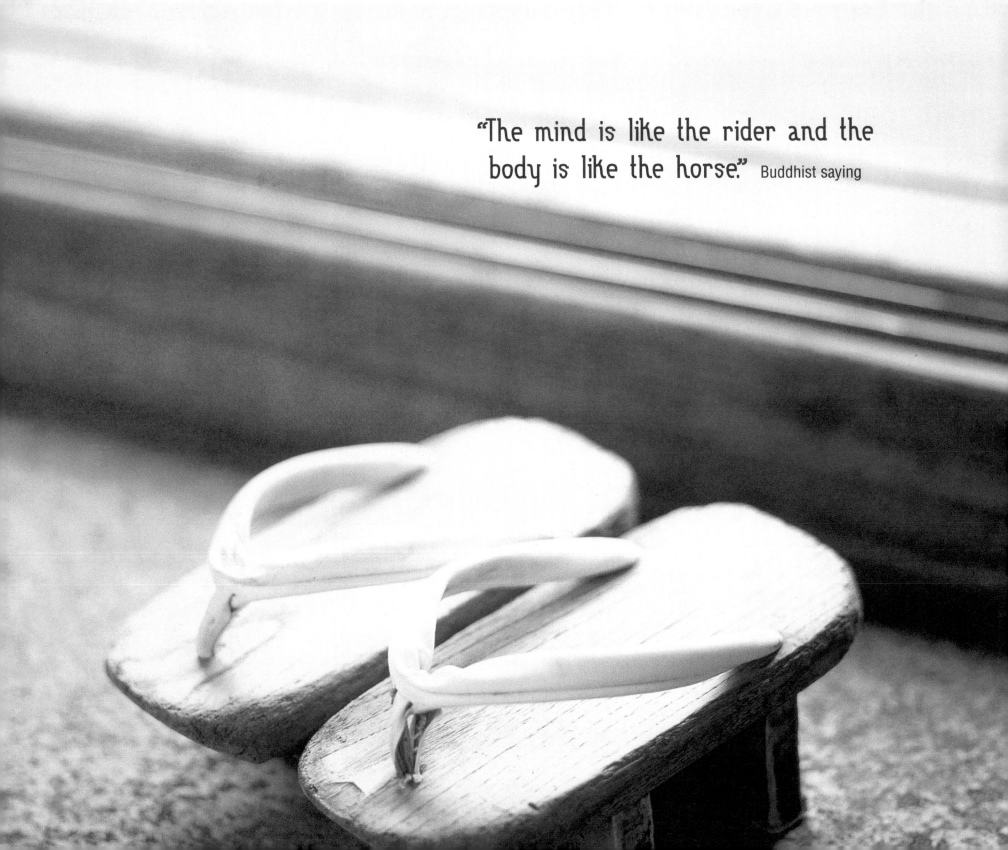

"The mind is like the rider and the body is like the horse." Buddhist saying

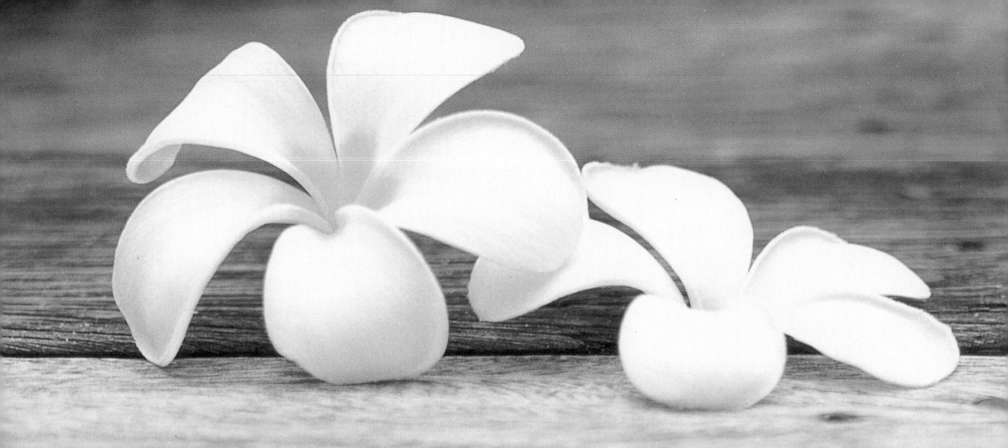

INSPIRATION FROM NATURE

Nature has a calming influence on the spirit. Simple pleasures such as breathing fresh air, feeling the sun on our skin and gazing at a beautiful landscape are natural restoratives. The sheer size of nature puts human problems in perspective. Think of the power of the ocean and the strength of a mountain. Many yoga postures emulate qualities of the natural world: Standing poses such as the "mountain pose" (see page 44) teach us the value of solidity and rootedness. Being at one with nature provides an antidote to the modern world in which we are surrounded by artificial devices such as computers and televisions. Nature sets the spirit free and allows us to feel connected to the universe.

Whenever you can, spend time in a natural environment: lie on your back on a patch of grass and gaze up at the clouds, go to a beach at night and watch the sea by moonlight, sit by a stream or river and absorb into your mind the sound of rushing water, climb a hill or a mountain simply to admire the view. If you live in town, be aware of the seasons and the signs of nature around you: birds nesting in the garden; plants and trees flourishing in the park; or a plant you have nurtured from seed gaining strength.

There are many ways to co-exist with nature. You could put a bird table outside your window, introduce rocks and plants to your workspace (see page 38) and conserve wild spaces in your garden. You could create your own sacred space using an arrangement of pebbles, rocks, shells, wood, a fountain or statue.

SPEND TIME IN NATURE

A peaceful way to spend time in nature is to practise a yoga exercise called *trataka*. This is a cleansing exercise for the eyes and facilitates a meditative state of mind. Sit in a meditative pose (see pages 80–1) and select a feature of the natural environment: a flower, tree, rock or the peak of a distant mountain; something that will remain still and is roughly at eye level. Focus on the feature with your eyes open. Keep gazing without blinking until your eyes start to fill with water. Now close your eyes and visualize the feature in your mind. Open your eyes again and continue to focus on the feature. Repeat this for several minutes.

BUDDHISM DERIVES MANY OF ITS TEACHINGS FROM THE NATURAL WORLD, WHICH CAN BE SUMMED UP AS:

There are no goals or ambitions in nature. The lives of plants and animals simply unfold with no special destination or purpose. The point of nature is simply to "be".

Nature provides excellent examples of "non-doing": day alternates with night, dormant trees come into bud, grow leaves and flowers, bear fruit and then shed their leaves and become dormant again. Stillness is as important as action.

Human life is not separate from the life of the environment. We are part of an interconnected whole. Nature provides our food, habitat and life-support. We are part of a vast natural cooperative.

There is no pressure of time in nature. Each organism operates according to its own rhythms and cycles. There is no such thing as going too slowly or too quickly.

Nature is playful, unpredictable, untameable. Hurricanes, volcanoes and earthquakes are not good or bad; they simply "are".

PEACE THROUGH MEDITATION

Meditation is a core part of most Eastern spiritual practices, but today many people in the West who meditate do so simply to relax. Western medicine acknowledges the importance of meditation for relieving stress, lowering blood pressure and enhancing general health and well-being. Whatever your reasons for meditating, the result will be the same: a greater sense of inner peace, serenity and harmony with the world around you.

In essence, meditation involves stilling the mind to stop the normal chatter of thoughts that accompanies you through your waking moments. Through meditation, this chatter is replaced by a state of unbroken consciousness in which you float with the stream of life. When you practise meditation, even for a short time, you'll start to appreciate the tranquil benefits it can bring.

Meditation usually begins as fleeting moments of concentration, often described as "gaps between thoughts". If you practise regularly, these gaps become longer. It can help to visualize your thoughts as waves – your aim is to extend the gap between the crest of one wave and the next. You must accept that when the waves come, you won't be swept away by them. The three most widely used methods are breath meditation, mantra (chanting)

meditation and meditating on an object such as a candle flame, or a mandala or yantra (visual symbols representing the universe). In each method, the breath, object or mantra is used simply as a prop that the mind can rest upon. Try the different methods until you find which one suits you best.

BREATH MEDITATION

You may already be familiar with the practice of focusing on your breath. During meditation, however, you concentrate on the rhythm of inhaling and exhaling without changing the quality or length of the breath. Breathe through your nose and make your awareness rest on the point inside your nostrils where the air first strikes. If your thoughts stray from your breath, gently but firmly guide them back. If it helps, try breath counting (see page 30).

MANTRA MEDITATION

Repeated sounds, or mantras, help to bring the mind into a meditative state. The single syllable "OM" is a sacred mantra, which is regarded in Hinduism as the sound of the universe. Use this or pick your own mantra such as "peace" or "one love", whatever is

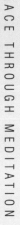

meaningful to you. Repeat your mantra aloud and concentrate on the vibrations of the sound throughout your mind, body and spirit. When your thoughts wander from your mantra, slowly but surely return them to the rhythmic sound you are making.

MEDITATING UPON AN OBJECT

Deep contemplation of an object can help you to focus inward and get into the right mental state for meditation. You can use any object, it needn't be a candle or symbolic item, but choose something with a clear shape or design that is not too distracting. Instead of actively looking at or thinking about the object, simply try to absorb its shape, colour or pattern into your mind and let your thoughts centre upon this. If you become distracted, use the object to centre yourself and draw your thoughts back in.

HOW TO START

Adepts at meditation can meditate anywhere at any time. However, when you first begin, try to make things as easy for yourself as possible by following a few simple guidelines. First, find a peaceful space, such as a bedroom or quiet park. Sit in a

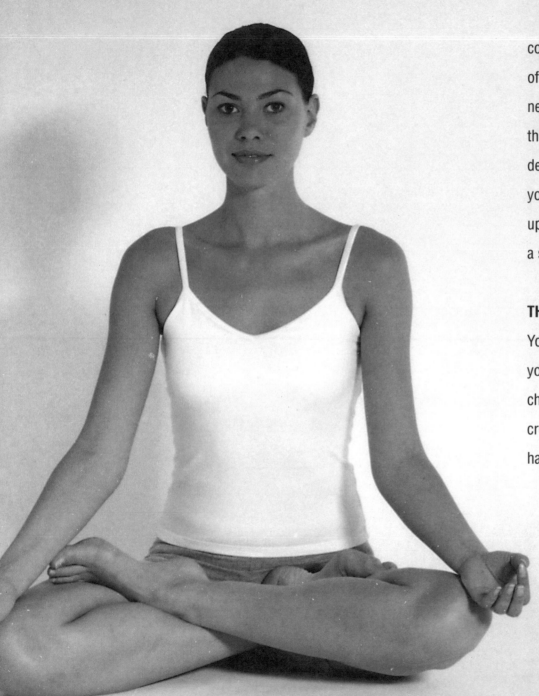

comfortable position – the poses shown on these pages are some of the best postures for meditation. If you're not comfortable, the needs of your body can be highly distracting. Focus your thoughts on your breath, mantra or object. If your thoughts wander, calmly and uncritically guide your mind back to the focus of your meditation. No matter how frequently the distractions pop up, reassure yourself that you are able to return your attention to a single point. Try to practise for 10 to 15 minutes at a time.

THE SITTING POSTURES

You need to be relaxed (but not sleepy) during meditation. Keep your spine straight and tall. If you prefer, sit in a straight-backed chair with your hands in your lap (see pages 44–5). Otherwise, sit cross-legged or choose one of the following positions. Rest your hands lightly on your knees, and make a circle with your thumb and forefinger if you like. If you are able to sit comfortably in the lotus position (shown opposite) this is the best one as it perfectly balances your body, but it is suitable only if you are very supple. Sit on the floor with your legs outstretched. Bend your left knee and lift the heel of your left foot to rest in your groin with the sole of the foot facing upward. Bend the right knee and lift your right foot, sole upturned, to rest in your groin.

A simpler version of this is the half-lotus. Sit on the floor with your legs outstretched. Bend your left knee and draw in the heel of your left foot to rest near your body. Bend your right knee and lift your right foot, sole upturned, to rest in your groin. Change the upper leg at each meditation session. Simpler still is the adept's pose (right). Sit on the floor with your legs outstretched. Cross your right foot in front of your body and bring your left foot in front of your right foot so that your heels are in alignment.

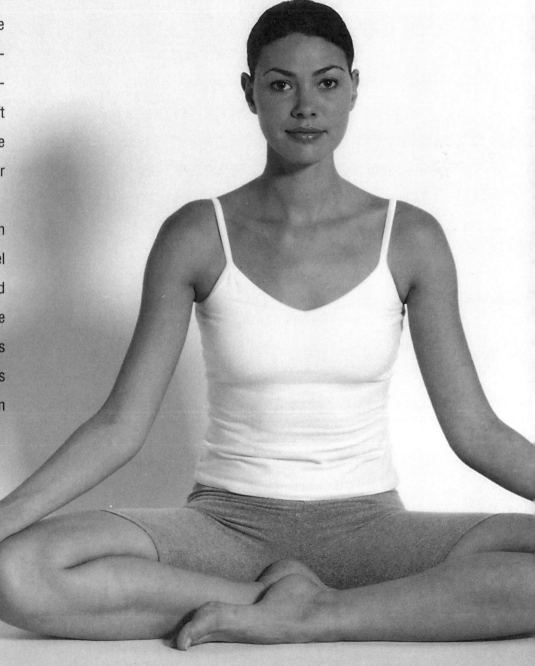

RELAX THROUGH BREATH

We have already been introduced to the profoundly relaxing benefits of breathing. However, as breathing is one of the most valuable tools you can use to influence your state of mind, it is worth spending time now exploring how breathing exercises can help you develop a sense of physical and emotional calm that you can carry with you throughout your life. By changing the way you breathe, you can slow your heart rate and lower your blood pressure. This helps you to relax and takes pressure off the cardio-vascular system – the part of the body most vulnerable to stress.

Eastern traditions emphasize the importance of deep breathing to the well-being of mind, body and spirit. In yoga, one of the core techniques is *pranayama* (breath control). The following breathing exercises are based on *pranayama* techniques. You can use these techniques whenever you need to relax but the best results happen when you practise them for their own sakes, every day. To enhance the relaxing effect, imagine all your stress and anxiety are melting away with each exhalation.

There is feedback between your brain and your breath. Feelings of excitement, anger and anxiety are accompanied by short, shallow, ragged breaths that penetrate only a little way into the lungs. In contrast, when you're relaxed, you take long, smooth breaths that flow deeply into the lungs. The following exercise will help you understand the connection between emotion and breath. Try it when you are in different states of mind.

If you are not used to regulating your breathing, aim to start gradually – the muscles of the respiratory system take time to become strong and supple. The golden rule is to breathe fluidly. If you get breathless during the exercises or feel that you are straining your lungs, you are trying too hard.

OBSERVE YOUR BREATHING

Sit in a cross-legged or other meditative position (see pages 80–1) and let yourself become aware of your breath. How does it feel? Is it smooth, slow and regular or rough, fast and uneven – or somewhere in between? Now place one hand on your abdomen and the other on your chest and note which part rises when you inhale? Compare your inhalations to your exhalations – is one shorter than the other or are they both of equal length? Observing your breathing habits teaches you breath awareness. You can then manipulate your breath to bring about relaxation.

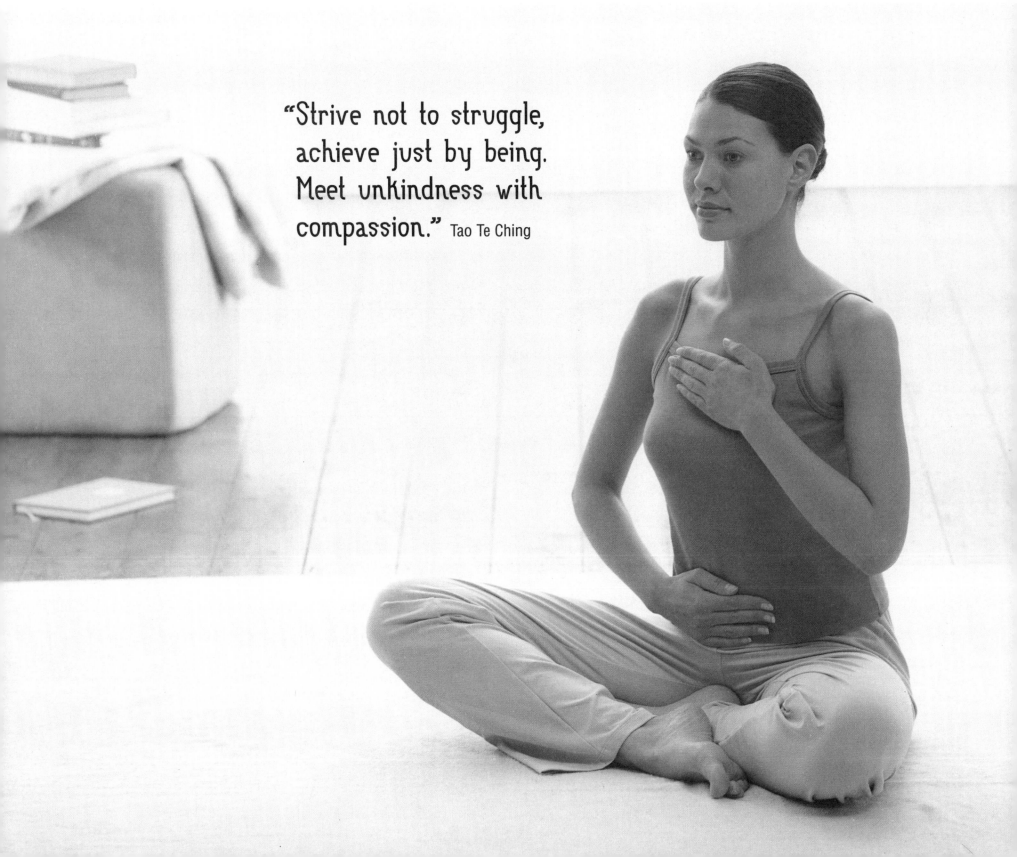

"Strive not to struggle, achieve just by being. Meet unkindness with compassion." Tao Te Ching

The most relaxing type of breath is one that is drawn down deeply. This is known as abdominal, qigong or *dan tien* breathing (see page 24). Although air does not literally go down as far as your abdomen, it moves into the deepest passages of your lungs, which pushes your diaphragm down and your abdomen out.

ABDOMINAL BREATHING

To practise abdominal breathing, sit as before with one hand on your chest and the other on your abdomen. Take a couple of normal breaths then inhale deeply through your nostrils. Let the air flow to the bottom of your lungs. Feel your diaphragm moving down and your belly pushing the palm of your lower hand out. Pause briefly, then exhale in one long, smooth breath. Feel your abdomen retract beneath your palm and your diaphragm move back to its resting position. Repeat this as often as you like.

An alternative method is to lie flat on your back with your legs a little way apart and your hands away from your body, palms up. Place a book on your abdomen, just below your navel and let your body sink into the floor. Now breathe deeply into your abdomen. Make the book rise and fall with each inhalation and exhalation. If

you feel dizzy, go back to your normal way of breathing and try again another day. If you practise abdominal breathing regularly, your respiratory system increases in strength and elasticity and any dizzy feelings will stop. You will also notice that deep breathing gives you an ongoing sense of poise and tranquillity.

Ideally, you should breathe deeply all the time. This is how you breathed as an infant and, unlike shallow chest breathing, it can enhance vitality, improve health and bring relaxation. Check your breathing regularly – if you find you are shallow breathing from the chest, make a conscious switch to abdominal breathing.

PRANIC BREATHING

A good way of summing up the technique of *pranic* breathing is "abdominal breathing plus imagination". As you inhale and exhale deeply into the abdomen, try to imagine that *prana* – the energy force that gives the spark of life to every living being – is feeding every part of your body. If it helps, stand tall and imagine the *prana* as coloured air that you are drawing up through the soles of your feet – on each inhalation the coloured air moves higher up into your body and diffuses to every single cell.

This exercise is particularly good at helping you to relax if you're suffering from tension in a particular part of your body. Using the power of your imagination, direct your breath to the area of tension. Imagine each inhalation sending warmth and healing to the area, and each exhalation taking away discomfort and tension. As you get more experienced at directing your breath in this way you'll find you can "breathe into" parts of the body that are remote from the lungs, such as the legs or the head.

EXTENDING THE BREATH

You can combine abdominal breathing with a relaxation technique known as "extending the breath". In *pranayama* the breath is divided into three stages: inhalation (*puraka*), retention (*kumbhaka*), and exhalation (*rechaka*). Each stage is associated with specific qualities: inhalation brings energy and vitality; retention (holding the breath before exhaling) allows the free flow of energy around the body; and exhalation is relaxing, grounding and cleansing. By increasing the length of your exhalation you can increase the relaxing effects of your breathing. Lengthening your exhalation has a tranquillizing effect on the mind and cleanses the body,

helping you to expel the stale, residual air that is otherwise left in the lungs. The more complete your exhalation, the greater the lung expansion and intake of air on your next inhalation.

Start by deliberately making your exhalations longer than your inhalations while you practise abdominal breathing. If you do this with your hand on your abdomen, you'll feel the strong upward pull of your diaphragm as you breathe out. Once you are comfortable with this technique, try holding your breath briefly after each exhalation (avoid holding your breath if you suffer from high blood pressure, lung or heart problems or you are pregnant).

Now combine these techniques by breathing in a ratio of 1:1:2. So, for example, inhale for a count of four, hold your breath for a count of four and then exhale to a count of eight.

You may find that rather than counting as you breathe it's easier to breathe to a silent repetition of the words *puraka*, *kumbhaka* and *rechaka*. To get the correct 1:1:2 ratio, you should inhale while saying *puraka* once, hold your breath while saying *kumbhaka* once and exhale to two repetitions of *rechaka*. Breathing to a strict ratio may be difficult at first – if so, just concentrate on making your exhalation longer than your inhalation.

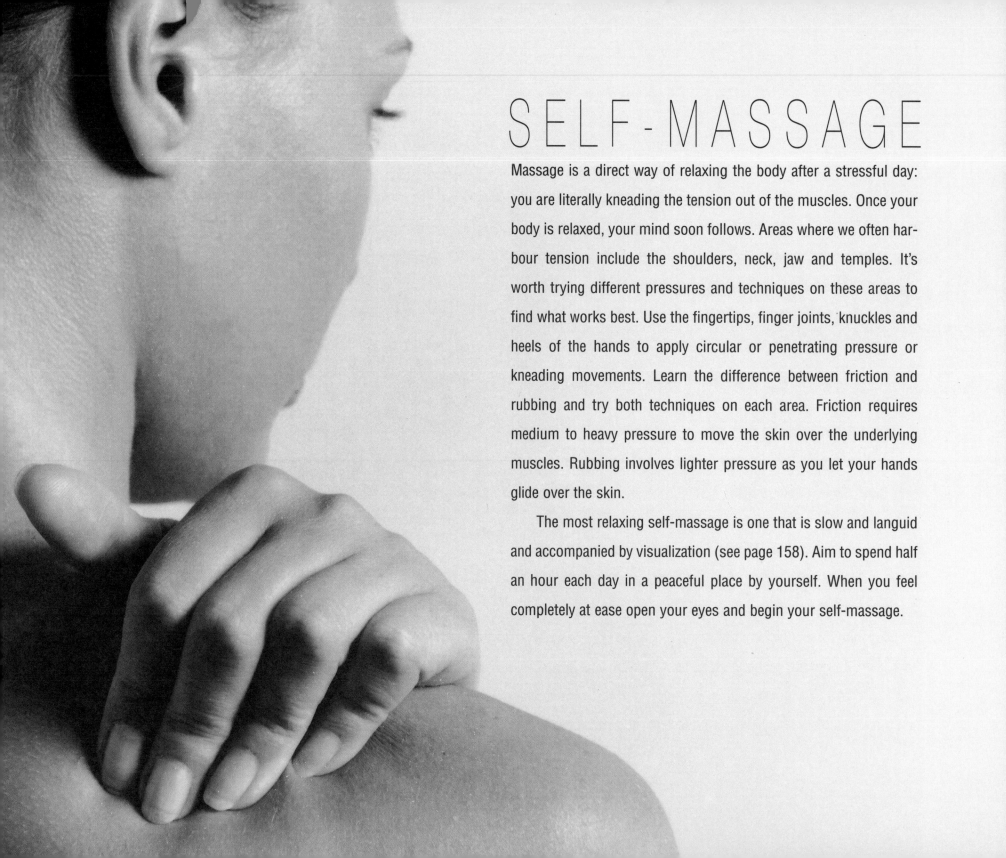

SELF-MASSAGE

Massage is a direct way of relaxing the body after a stressful day: you are literally kneading the tension out of the muscles. Once your body is relaxed, your mind soon follows. Areas where we often harbour tension include the shoulders, neck, jaw and temples. It's worth trying different pressures and techniques on these areas to find what works best. Use the fingertips, finger joints, knuckles and heels of the hands to apply circular or penetrating pressure or kneading movements. Learn the difference between friction and rubbing and try both techniques on each area. Friction requires medium to heavy pressure to move the skin over the underlying muscles. Rubbing involves lighter pressure as you let your hands glide over the skin.

The most relaxing self-massage is one that is slow and languid and accompanied by visualization (see page 158). Aim to spend half an hour each day in a peaceful place by yourself. When you feel completely at ease open your eyes and begin your self-massage.

SHOULDER KNEADING (Left)

Bend your arm and take hold of your opposite shoulder. Massage the muscles at the back of the shoulder by applying deep circular pressure with your fingertips. Work your way along from the neck to the top of the arm. Concentrate on knotted areas. Repeat on the other side.

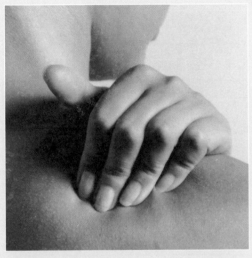

NECK KNEADING (Right)

Bend your arm and place your fingertips on the opposite side of your neck toward the back. Apply circular or static fingertip pressure to the muscles in this area starting at the base of the neck and moving up to the base of the skull and down again. Repeat on the other side.

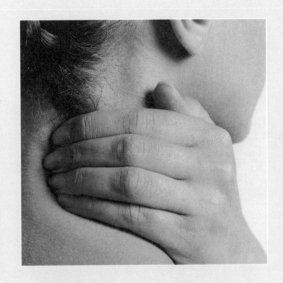

JAW CIRCLING (Left)

To locate your jaw muscles, place your hands on your cheeks and open your mouth wide and shut it again – you will feel them moving. Now, with your jaw relaxed, press your fingertips into your jaw muscles and move them in large slow circles, first clockwise then anticlockwise.

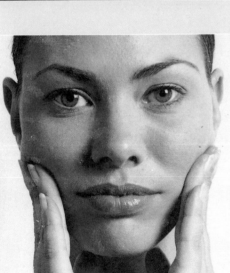

TEMPLE CIRCLING (Right)

Place the fingertips of your index and middle fingers on your temples, apply medium pressure and move your fingers in slow circles, first clockwise then anticlockwise.

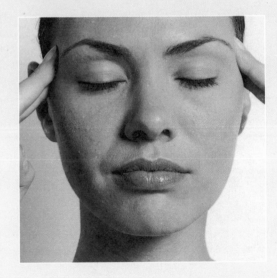

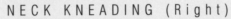

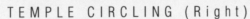

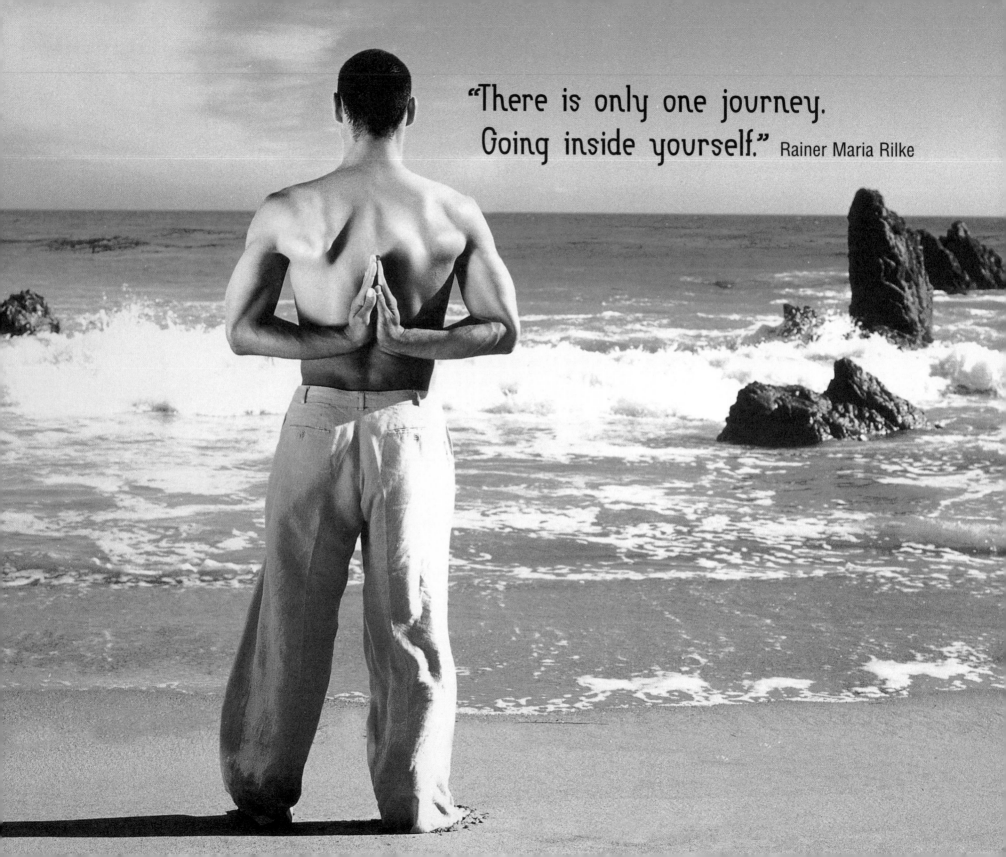

"There is only one journey.
Going inside yourself." Rainer Maria Rilke

MOVEMENT AND RELEASE

Many of us associate "relaxing" with sitting still, for example, when lounging in front of the television, sitting in the garden or lying on the beach. But deep relaxation is often best achieved through movement. As we stretch our muscles we release the pockets of tension that otherwise prevent us achieving the calm we seek. We can then focus inward and spend a few minutes inside ourselves rather than in the chaotic outside world. The steps on pages 92 and 93 ease muscular tension through yoga movements. As you practise these poses, enhance their beneficial effects by drawing together what you have learnt elsewhere in this chapter. Be aware ("mindful") of your movements, focus on your breathing and use visualization to feel the tension leaving you.

RELIEVING TENSION THROUGH POSTURES

Before you start, warm up with a few rounds of the suppleness sequence on pages 52–5. If you find any of them difficult or uncomfortable, take them more slowly. Don't push yourself beyond your natural limits; the aim is to release tension rather than to exert force. Let your body sink deeply into each pose. Stay in each posture for as long as is comfortable – aim to hold for

three to five deep breaths, if possible. Spend as long as you like in the final resting pose – this is known as the "corpse pose" because the body lies as still and quiet as a corpse. It is the classic relaxation posture in yoga and, because your body is motionless, it gives you the opportunity to observe your state of mind. Listen to your thoughts. Are they peaceful, restless, agitated or sluggish? Whatever the state of your thoughts, try to judge them impartially rather than being preoccupied or swept away by them.

Breathe deeply and steadily through your nose and try to coincide the inhalations with upward or forward movements, and the exhalations with downward movements. Concentrate on the breath flowing smoothly in and out of your body. Take your breath down deeply so you can feel your abdomen expanding and relaxing with each breath. Keep returning your attention to your breath – this is the key to inducing mental stillness and calm. Say to yourself: "I know I am breathing in, I know I am breathing out."

As you relax in each pose, mentally scan your body for pockets of tension. The areas where it's common to hold muscle tension are the face, jaw, neck, shoulders and back. Each time you exhale, imagine the tension is floating or melting away.

YOGA POSTURES DISSOLVE MUSCLE TENSION AND AID RELAXATION THROUGH THE MOVEMENT OF MUSCLES. TRY TO PRACTISE THIS SEQUENCE EACH DAY.

BE MINDFUL OF YOUR BODY AND THE WAY IT MOVES. FOCUS ON YOUR BREATH AND, WHEN YOU EXHALE, IMAGINE ALL TENSION MELTING AWAY.

RELAXING YOGA SEQUENCE

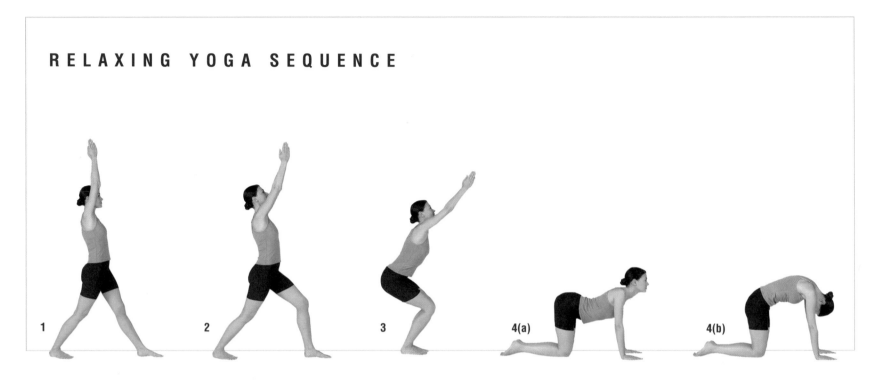

1 Stand with your legs wide apart and your arms by your sides. Turn your right foot in slightly, turn your left foot out at right angles and swivel your body from the hips to face in the direction of your left foot (keep your right leg straight). Bring your arms together above your head so your palms are touching.

2 Bend your left knee so it is directly above your left ankle and your calf is vertical. Look up at your palms and breathe deeply. Slowly come out of the posture. Repeat on the other side.

3 Stand with your feet together. Lift your arms up alongside your ears and place your palms together. Look up at your hands and then bend your legs as if you are going to sit down on a chair. Draw up your pelvic floor and abdominal muscles to support the pose. Gently return to standing.

4 (a) Come down to the floor and adopt an all-fours position. Keep your back parallel to the floor and your head and neck in line with your back. Now inhale, hollow your back and lift your head and buttocks as high as you can. (b) On an exhalation, arch your spine upward and lower your head down between your arms. Tuck your buttocks in and pull your abdominal muscles in toward your spine.

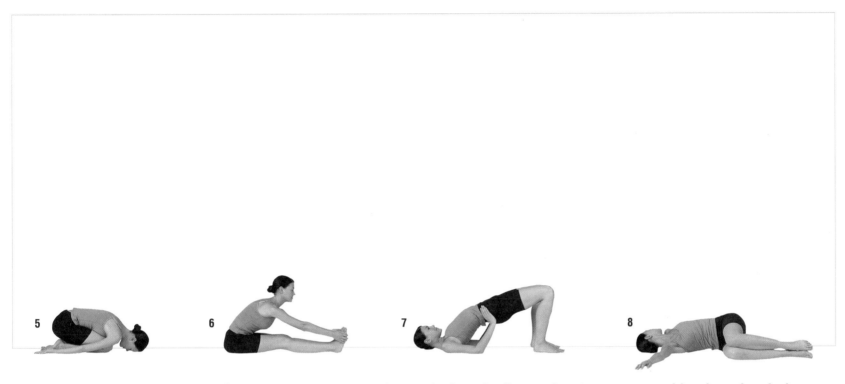

5 Come into a kneeling position. Gently lower your head and upper body to the floor and rest your arms and hands, palms facing up, alongside your body. Let your body relax completely into the pose.

6 Sit on the floor with your legs out in front of you and your feet flexed. Raise your arms over your head and lengthen your spine. Fold forward at your hips as far as you can, keeping your back flat. Clasp your legs or feet. Try to elongate your spine on each inhalation. Bring your body closer to your legs on each exhalation. Keep the natural curve in your lower back.

7 Lie on your back with your knees bent and your feet in line with your buttocks. Gently raise your hips and spine off the ground. Support your lower back with your palms and push your chest up high. Don't let your knees move apart.

8 Lie on your back with your knees close to your chest and your arms out to the sides at shoulder level. Gently drop your knees to the floor on the right side and turn your head to look at your left shoulder. Hold this twist for a few breaths. Repeat on the other side. To finish, lie flat on your back with your legs a little way apart and your hands away from your body, palms facing up. This is the corpse pose. Let your entire body sink into the floor. Close your eyes and focus on your breathing.

LEARN TO LISTEN

OBSERVE, DON'T JUDGE

CONSIDER OTHERS

"Lying down on the ground like a corpse removes fatigue and brings rest to the mind."

Hatha Yoga Pradipika

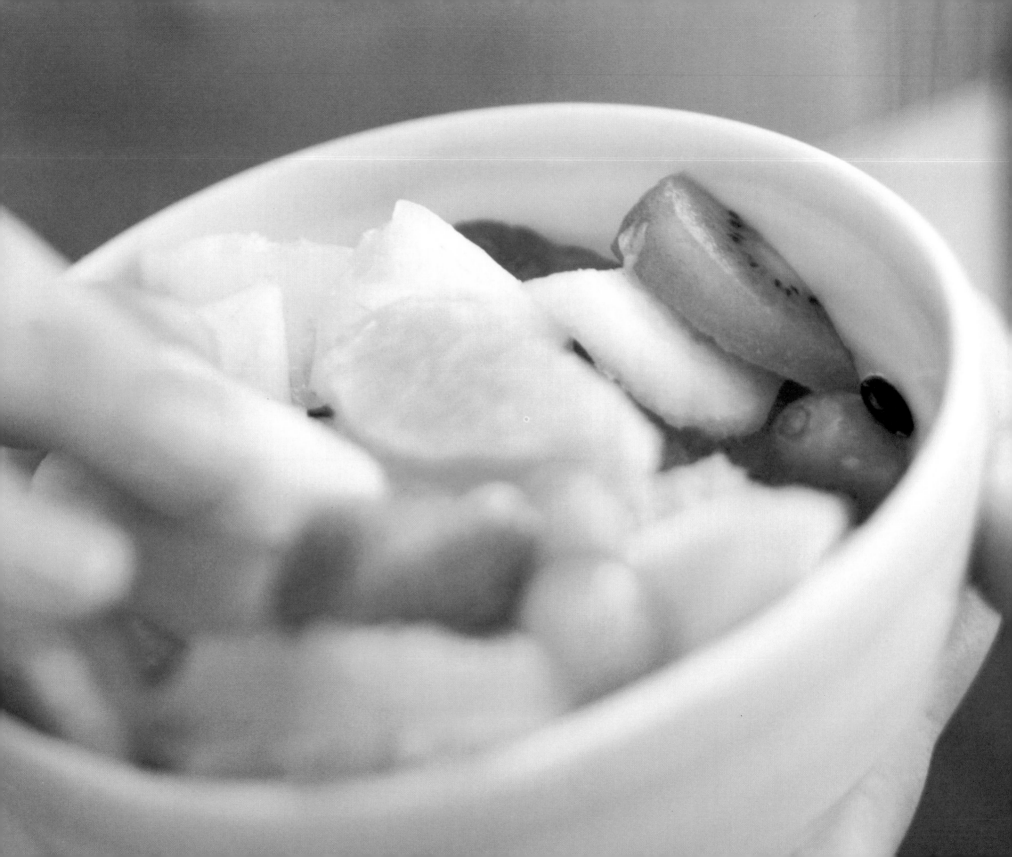

EATING & DRINKING

In the East it is accepted that to attain life-long health and well-being you should eat wholesome foods, drink pure fluids and take time to enjoy meals. Yet many in the West avoid natural foods in favour of processed meals that are high in calories and low in vital nutrients, leading to high rates of diet-related diseases.

This chapter offers suggestions about how to incorporate the healthy principles of traditional and Eastern diets into your life. It also discusses ways to improve the way you eat and digest food through techniques such as mindfulness and yoga.

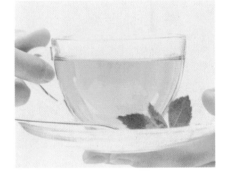

HEALTHY EATING

Nutritionists say the ideal diet for long-term health is one based on unrefined complex carbohydrates (starchy foods), complemented by lots of fresh fruit and vegetables. However, the typical Western diet comprises foods that are processed, high in added sugar and salt (see page 102) and saturated fat, and low in fibre, essential fats, vitamins and minerals. This diet is implicated in obesity, diabetes, cancer and diseases of the heart and colon.

In Eastern countries people still rely heavily on carbohydrate foods such as rice, lentils and soya (see page 104). The Hunza people of Kashmir – who are famous for their longevity and freedom from disease – live on a diet of whole grains, fresh fruit and vegetables, goat's milk and natural drinking water. Traditional diets also have other things in common: foods are natural, fresh, and tend to include less meat than we eat in the West.

EAT NATURAL

Aim to eat foods that are as close to their natural state as possible. For example, eat wholegrain bread and flour, and brown rice – their heavily processed white equivalents lack valuable fibre and nutrients. Avoid – or limit – convenience food, such as crisps, cakes, biscuits, high-sugar snacks, prepared meals and fast-food. If you have a sweet tooth, make cakes and cookies at home using wholefood ingredients, and use honey as a sweetener rather than refined white sugar. Keep your body hydrated with natural fluids such as plain water (see page 118), fresh fruit juice (see page 122) or herbal teas rather than sugary or caffeinated drinks such as fruit drinks, squash, cola, tea and coffee.

EAT FRESH

Whenever possible, eat the freshest food you can find. According to yogic teaching, food is richest in life-force energy (*prana*) when it is newly picked. If you can't grow your own produce, eat food that looks, smells, feels and tastes fresh. Choose fresh food in preference to canned, bottled, salted, or irradiated food. Valuable nutrients, including enzymes, phytochemicals and antioxidant vitamins (all of which help protect against disease), are damaged or even destroyed by cooking, so it makes sense to eat lots of uncooked foods. Snack on raw fruit and vegetables such as apples, apricots, berries, citrus fruit, grapes, pears, carrots, celery, radishes, peppers, spinach, tomatoes and watercress.

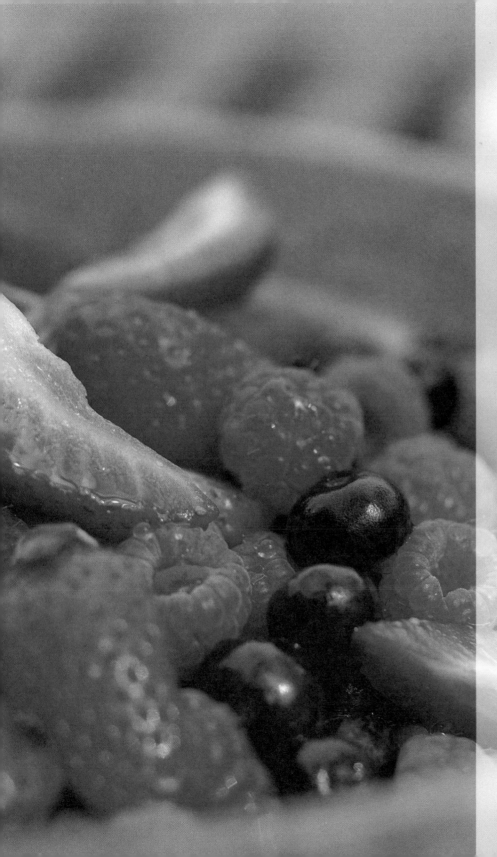

EAT LESS MEAT

It is a myth that you need to eat meat to get sufficient protein to stay healthy. Diets that contain little or no meat can also provide enough protein for your needs. For example, the combination of lentils and rice (as in the Indian dish *khichuri*; see page 103) provides a good source of protein; so do tofu, beans, seeds and nuts. There are sound health reasons for eating a diet that is based on plant foods. Meat can be high in saturated fat, which is linked to heart disease. Plant foods, however, are naturally low in saturated fat and high in vitamins, minerals and complex carbohydrates.

In yoga teachings on diet (see page 114) plant foods are said to have greater life-promoting properties than meat because plants receive nourishment directly from the sun, the source of energy for the whole planet. Eating plant foods enables us to access this energy in the most direct way possible. Meat is a third-hand source of energy and therefore less beneficial.

If you choose not to eat meat or fish, make sure your diet includes a wide variety of plant sources of proteins so that you get all the essential amino acids (the basic building blocks that make up the proteins in your body) that you need for optimum health.

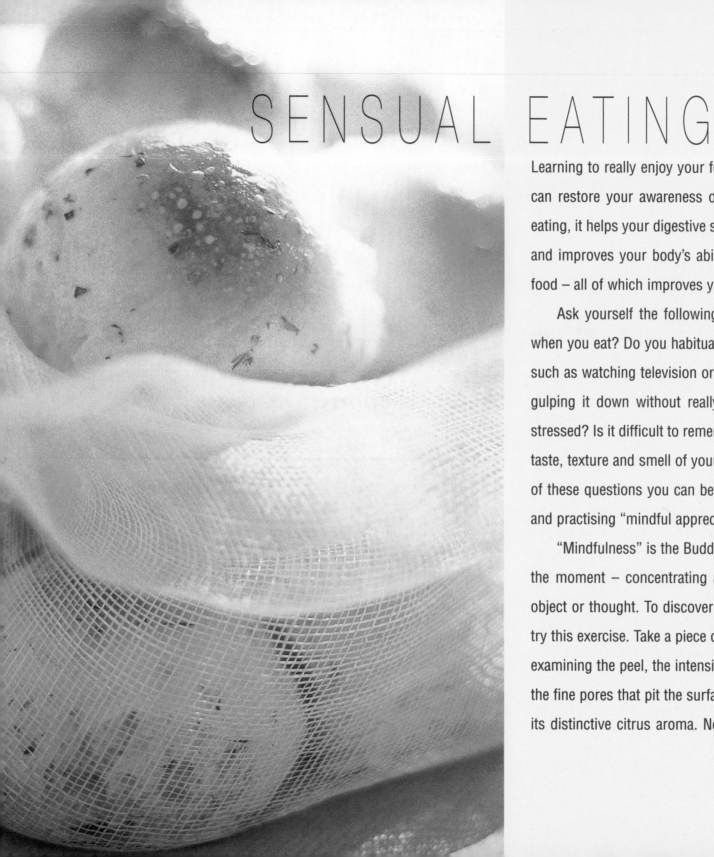

SENSUAL EATING

Learning to really enjoy your food can bring amazing benefits. It can restore your awareness of the simple, sensual pleasure of eating, it helps your digestive system to function more efficiently, and improves your body's ability to extract nutrients from your food – all of which improves your general health and well-being.

Ask yourself the following questions. Are you preoccupied when you eat? Do you habitually eat while doing something else such as watching television or working? Do you rush your food, gulping it down without really tasting it, or eat when tired or stressed? Is it difficult to remember the last time you relished the taste, texture and smell of your food? If you answer "yes" to any of these questions you can benefit by changing the way you eat and practising "mindful appreciation" during eating.

"Mindfulness" is the Buddhist concept of being immersed in the moment – concentrating all your attention on one activity, object or thought. To discover mindful appreciation for yourself, try this exercise. Take a piece of fruit such as an orange. Start by examining the peel, the intensity of its colour and the delicacy of the fine pores that pit the surface. As you peel the orange, inhale its distinctive citrus aroma. Now divide the flesh into individual segments. Feel the texture of the pith and skin with your fingers and tongue. Nibble a hole in a segment and taste the juice. How would you describe it to someone who's never tasted an orange? Sweet, refreshing, cold, acidic? Now put the piece in your mouth and concentrate on the texture and taste as you chew. Imagine the tree on which the orange grew. Through mindfulness, you will gain maximum satisfaction from everything you see and do.

CHANGE YOUR EATING PATTERN

Before each meal, turn off the television so you can devote yourself to the pleasures of eating and spend a few moments observing the sensual qualities of the food. Look at and smell your food before you take the first mouthful – it is the sight and smell of food that first stimulate the appetite and cause the digestive juices to flow (think of the delicious aroma of freshly baked bread).

Be aware of the way in which your body is receiving food. Are you calm, relaxed and sitting up straight so that food can move easily through your digestive system, or are you stressed and hunched up so that your stomach and intestines are compressed? Try consciously to relax your body (always stay upright)

and take a few deep breaths between each mouthful – observe whether this enhances your appreciation of food.

As well as considering how you eat, think about when you eat. You are probably conditioned to believe that you should eat three meals a day – say, at breakfast, lunch and dinner – a pattern that fits conveniently into the standard working day. Yet it makes more sense to feed the body when it asks for food. So, try to become attuned to your natural hunger signals. Before a meal, ask yourself whether you are hungry or whether you are eating out of habit – by practising mindful appreciation you encourage this kind of awareness. Start feeding yourself only when you need to. You can still have three meals a day if you want to, but aim to eat less at each meal and graze on healthy snacks in between.

Another natural signal to be more aware of is satiety. Stop part of the way through a meal and ask yourself whether you want to continue eating. Notice the difference between continuing to eat out of hunger and continuing to eat for other reasons – emotional gratification, for example. If you usually eat every morsel on the plate, leave some food behind. Ask yourself an hour later whether you have really missed that food.

EASTERN HERBS & SPICES

The Western diet relies heavily on salt and sugar to flavour food, not just in tinned and ready-made meals, but also bread, breakfast cereals, yogurts and fruit drinks. In the long term, excess salt and sugar are bad for health – leading to high blood pressure, obesity, heart disease and adult-onset diabetes. Food manufacturers also use artificial flavourings and flavour enhancers, such as monosodium glutamate (MSG) in food which, even though their effects are not completely understood, are not thought to make a positive contribution to the diet.

The best way to avoid excess salt and sugar and artificial flavouring is to cook your own meals using healthy ingredients; this way you know exactly what you are eating. Some of the most flavoursome recipes come from the East. Rather than relying on salt and sugar for flavour, Eastern recipes use aromatic herbs and spices, now readily available in Western supermarkets.

These flavourings not only make food taste good but they also have health benefits. Garlic, ginger and chillies can prevent abnormal blood clotting and so help guard against cardiovascular disease; garlic also has anti-cancer properties. Cinnamon, cardamom, cumin, coriander and mustard seeds stimulate the appetite and enhance digestion. Cloves have antiseptic properties, and sesame contains essential fatty acids that lower the level of "bad" cholesterol in the blood and so keep the heart healthy.

TIPS ON EASTERN FLAVOURING

You don't have to adopt a completely new cuisine. Here are a few simple ideas for incorporating Eastern flavourings into your diet:

- Stir-fry vegetables in your own combination of spices – ginger, garlic, mustard seeds and chilli, for example.
- Add crushed garlic and finely chopped spring onion, or crushed mustard seeds and finely chopped chilli to mashed potato.
- Fry broccoli or Brussels sprouts in sesame oil and/or sprinkle them with sesame seeds.
- Add a little raw, finely chopped chilli to salad dressings.
- Add a pinch of cumin, and some finely chopped coriander and chilli to scrambled eggs.
- Tie cloves and crushed cardamom pods in a muslin bag and use to flavour rice pudding or cooked fruit such as apricots.
- Add cinnamon or grated ginger to cooked apples or apple pie.
- Flavour tea with cloves and cinnamon sticks.

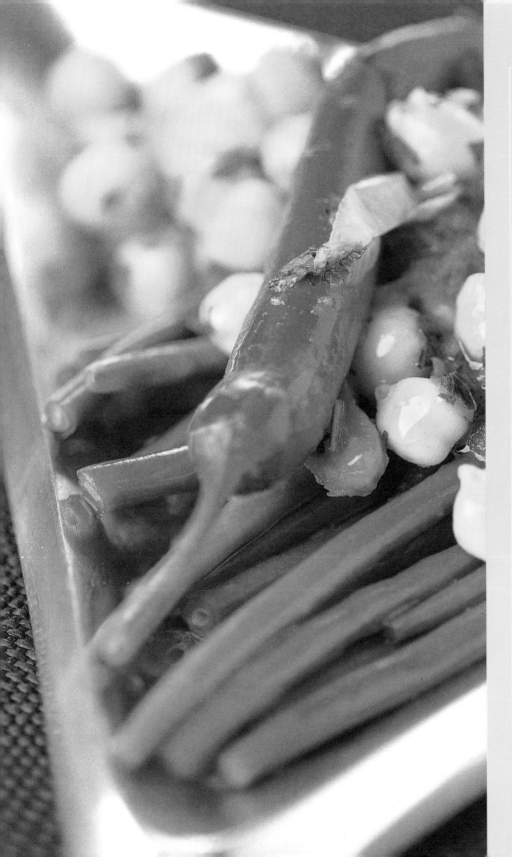

SPICY CHICKPEAS

This simple dish is a great way to use garlic, ginger, chilli, cumin and coriander – all popular Eastern flavourings – to best aromatic effect. Serve the chickpeas with lightly steamed, fresh, green beans and basmati rice cooked with red lentils (this is called *khichuri* in India).

SERVES 4

2 tablespoons extra virgin olive oil

1 teaspoon ground cumin

1 teaspoon ground coriander seeds

2 cloves garlic

1 onion, chopped

450 g/1 lb/2 cups cooked chickpeas

6 tomatoes, skinned and chopped

1 teaspoon dried thyme

Pinch of chilli pepper

1 teaspoon fresh, grated ginger

100 ml/3½ fl oz/½ cup water or vegetable stock

Sea salt and pepper

Heat the oil gently in a large saucepan or wok. Add the cumin, coriander, garlic and onion. Stir-fry for 3–4 minutes, add the chickpeas, and then the rest of the ingredients. Bring to the boil and simmer gently for 15 minutes, adding a little extra water from time to time if necessary. Add seasoning, according to taste, and serve.

EASTERN STAPLE FOODS

The Eastern diet is high in unrefined cereals and pulses, such as rice, noodles, soya beans and lentils, all of which are renowned for their health-giving properties. There is now consensus among nutritionists that a diet based on these kinds of complex carbohydrate foods is important for good health and well-being and can help guard against disease – yet most people in the West don't eat nearly enough of them. Unprocessed carbohydrates contain high amounts of fibre, which helps to prevent cardiovascular disease, bowel cancer and diabetes. Whenever possible, try to include the following foods in your diet – ideally they should make up 50 per cent of your daily calorie intake.

RICE AND NOODLES

Rice is the staple cereal that is eaten in the East. Brown rice is particularly nutritious because it retains the fibre and nutrients, such as thiamin (Vitamin B$_1$), that are lost during the refining and milling of white rice. Brown rice helps to maintain the health of the gut, it stabilizes blood sugar levels and is an excellent alternative to wheat for those who suffer from gluten intolerance. Thiamin is vital for healthy muscles and nerves.

Noodles are widely eaten in countries such as China and Japan. Japanese soba noodles, which are made from buckwheat flour, are a valuable part of a wholefood diet. Buckwheat is an unrefined grain that is a good source of vegetable protein and minerals. Buckwheat also contains a substance called rutin, which is good for the health of the heart and blood vessels.

SOYA BEANS AND OTHER PULSES

Soya beans yield an amazing array of food products, including miso, tempeh, tofu, soya milk, soya flour and soy sauce. Soya beans are an excellent source of plant protein (in China soya is known as "meat without bones") and also contain iron, calcium, potassium, magnesium, folic acid and essential fatty acids.

Soya products are good for a healthy heart and digestive system and provide a great alternative to animal products if you are vegetarian or trying to cut down on your meat consumption. Soya beans are rich in plant oestrogens, which can relieve menstrual and menopausal symptoms and help to prevent breast cancer. The healthiest soya products to include in your diet are tofu, soya milk and soya flour. Avoid genetically modified soya.

COCONUT DHAL

Dhal is a delicious way of using lentils and is also cheap and nutritious. There are many ways of making dhal – this recipe includes the delicate taste of coconut milk. Serve as a starter or as a side dish.

SERVES 4

2 tablespoons vegetable oil

5 shallots, finely chopped

½ teaspoon ground turmeric

4 cloves garlic, finely chopped

1 small cinnamon stick

2 red chillies, finely chopped

180 g/6 oz/1 cup red lentils, washed

1 teaspoon salt

600 ml/1 pint vegetable stock

300 ml/½ pint coconut milk

1 tablespoon fresh lemon juice

Freshly ground black pepper

Heat the oil gently in a large saucepan. Fry the shallots for 3 minutes and then add the turmeric, garlic, cinnamon stick and chillies and fry for a further minute, stirring continuously. Stir the lentils into the pan and add the salt and stock. Leave to simmer for 45 minutes or until the lentils are cooked. Stir in the coconut milk and cook for a further 10 minutes. Add the lemon juice and black pepper and serve.

The lentil is another major ingredient in the Eastern diet. Two common types of lentils are brown (actually brownish-green) lentils and red lentils. Red lentils can be bought whole or split, although the split kind, which you don't need to soak, is the most readily available in the West. Lentils are rich in protein, potassium, iron, calcium and folic acid, and they can help to stabilize blood sugar levels, prevent heart disease and lower levels of "bad" cholesterol (low-density lipoproteins) in the blood.

You can make beans and other pulses, including whole lentils, tastier and more easily digestible by allowing them to germinate and produce sprouts, which turns their starch into sugar. There are different methods of preparation according to the type of pulse. For lentils, soak in lukewarm water for 12 hours (changing the water after 8 hours), drain, and place between layers of damp kitchen paper. Leave the lentils in a dark place, such as a turned-off oven, keeping them damp at all times. After 36 hours you should see small sprouts developing. Wash the lentils and discard any loose skins. Store the sprouted lentils in a sealed container in the refrigerator for up to a week. To cook the lentils, stir-fry or boil for 3–4 minutes or steam for 6–8 minutes.

COOKING THE EASTERN WAY

One of the most important pieces of equipment that is used in Eastern cooking is a thin-walled bowl-shaped metal pan. In India and Pakistan this pan is called a "karahi" but in the West it is more widely known by its Chinese name of "wok". The round-bottomed shape allows heat to spread quickly and evenly over the surface so that the food cooks rapidly, thus sealing in nutrients and flavour. The speed of cooking also helps to conserve scarce fuel.

The wok is now popular in the West, but few Westerners use the pan to its full potential. In China, the wok is used for stir-frying, deep frying, boiling, stewing and steaming. Stir-frying and steaming are healthy cooking methods because they retain most of the nutrients and require little or no oil. If you don't own a wok you can stir-fry in a frying pan and steam foods over a saucepan.

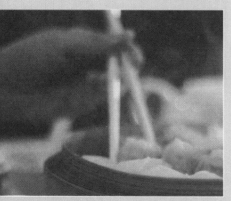

STIR-FRYING

To prepare for stir-frying, cut food into bite-sized pieces. Suitable foods include tender cuts of meat such as chicken or sirloin beef, fish, shellfish and vegetables. Heat a small amount of oil in a wok – just enough to coat the inside of the pan. Choose an oil such as sunflower, peanut, soybean or corn oil that can withstand high temperatures (never use butter). Keep stirring the food during cooking. This quickly seals the food and prevents the absorption of excess fat. The result is food that is crunchy (in the case of vegetables) and flavoursome while also being low in fat.

STEAMING

Steamed food cooks quickly and easily with no extra fat and preserves most of the water-soluble vitamins such as B-complex and C (boiling, in contrast, depletes foods of water-soluble vitamins). Steamed food is succulent and tender and also looks attractive because it keeps its shape during cooking. Steaming is an ideal way to cook fish, shellfish, chicken and vegetables.

The traditional way to steam food in a wok is to place a stack of bamboo steamers above simmering water or stock (this is how the Chinese steam rice). Make sure that the food is not packed too tightly so the steam can circulate freely. If the liquid boils away, always replace it with boiling water. Western-style steamers – pots with compartments to hold the food – are also available.

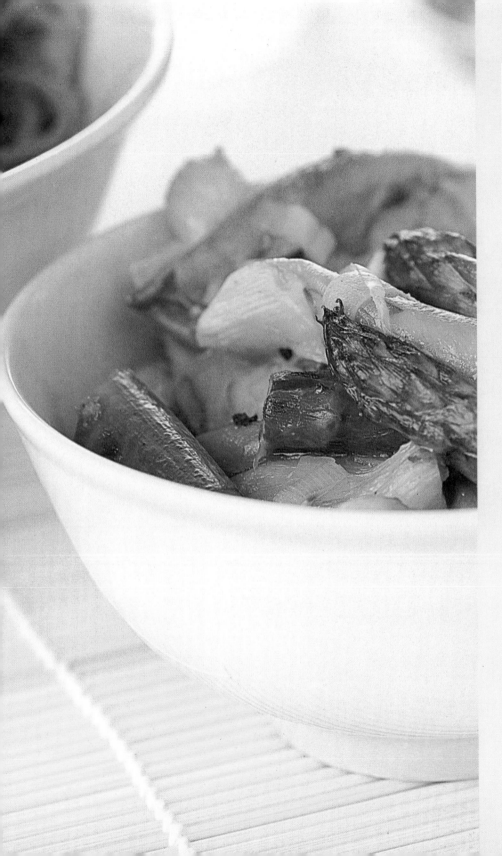

ASPARAGUS, TOFU AND MUSHROOMS

This is a classic Chinese stir-fry recipe that is traditionally cooked in a wok. You can always substitute your own choice of vegetables if you wish. Serve at once with a portion of cooked noodles.

SERVES 4

2 tablespoons extra virgin olive oil

225 g/8 oz/1 cup tofu (bean curd), diced

1 small leek, sliced

225 g/8 oz/1 cup oyster mushrooms, cleaned and left whole

1 clove garlic, crushed; 1 teaspoon fresh ginger, finely chopped

1 bunch green asparagus, cut into small pieces (discard the
    bottom 2 in/5 cm of the stalks)

100 ml/3½ fl oz /½ cup vegetable stock or water

2 tablespoons soy sauce; 2 tablespoons dry sherry

1 teaspoon cornflour, dissolved in a little warm water

Heat the oil in a wok or large frying pan and stir-fry the tofu for a couple of minutes. Add the leek and stir for another minute, then the mushrooms, garlic and ginger, stir-frying until the mushrooms release their moisture. Add the asparagus, stock, soy sauce and sherry, then cover and simmer very gently until the asparagus is tender. Add the cornflour and stir until the sauce thickens.

YIN AND YANG FOODS

In Chinese medicine it is believed that, to achieve health and bodily harmony, you must balance your intake of cool, bland foods full of *yin* energy with hot, spicy foods full of *yang* energy. The concept of *yin* and *yang* are fundamental to Chinese thinking. Everything in the universe can be ascribed *yin* and *yang* qualities: *yin* is characterized as dark, cold, night and female, while *yang* is light, hot, day and male. Each is opposite but complementary to the other. When you eat the correct balance of foods your own *yin* and *yang* will be balanced and energy (*chi* or *qi*) will flow unimpeded through your body, enhancing your health and well-being.

THE YIN-YANG DIET

In general, your diet should include neutral foods, such as plain rice, in combination with a balance of *yin* and *yang* foods. To observe the principles of a *yin* and *yang* diet, you should tailor your diet to your constitution. An excess of *yin* or *yang* leads to overweight; a deficiency of *yin* or *yang* leads to underweight.

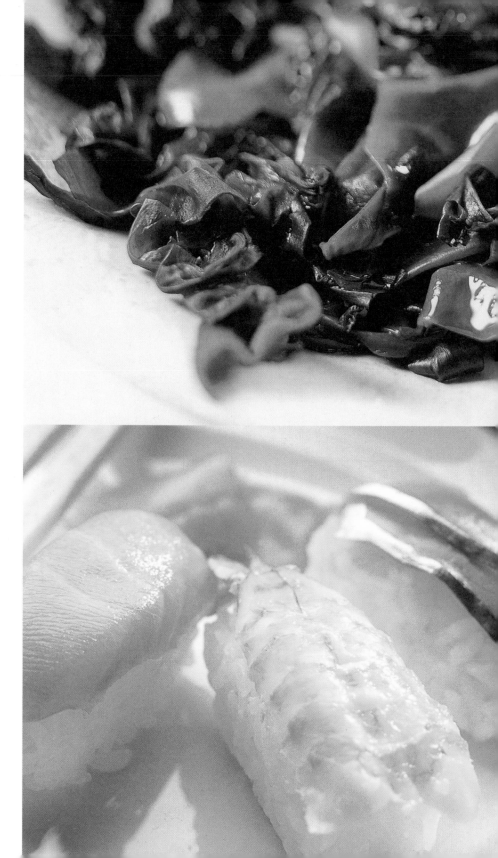

STUFFED MUSHROOMS

This recipe shows how a *yin* food (mushrooms) can be combined with *yang* foods (garlic, shallots and soy sauce) to create a balanced dish. This dish can be served as a starter, a vegetable accompaniment or a vegetarian main course.

SERVES 4

12–16 large, flat mushrooms

3 tablespoons extra virgin olive oil

2 cloves garlic, finely chopped

1 shallot, finely chopped

1 sprig fresh (or ½ teaspoon dried) rosemary, chopped

1 tablespoon soy sauce

4–5 tablespoons breadcrumbs

1 small bunch parsley, finely chopped

Remove the mushroom stalks and set aside. Scoop out the black gills inside the mushroom caps and discard. Place the caps hollow side upward in an oiled ovenproof dish or baking tray. Finely chop the mushroom stalks and sauté in olive oil for one minute. Add the garlic and shallot and heat through. Stir in the rosemary and soy sauce and simmer until the mushroom stalks release their moisture. Add enough breadcrumbs to soak up the liquid, then remove from the heat and add the parsley. Fill the mushroom caps with mixture. Bake for 5–10 minutes at 400°F/200°C/gas mark 6 until golden brown.

People with an excess of *yin* tend to be short of breath, slow moving, heavy sleepers and prone to fluid retention and cold extremities. They should try to cut down on *yin* foods and include more *yang* foods. Individuals with an excess of *yang* tend to sweat excessively, feel hot and be prone to hyperactivity, overeating and drinking. They should eat more *yin* foods and fewer *yang* foods.

Yin foods tend to be cooling, watery, soft and dark in colour. Aquatic animals and plants such as fish and seaweed are *yin*; so are foods that grow underground or in darkness, such as root vegetables or mushrooms. *Yin* foods include barley, oats, wheat, aubergine, beansprouts, beetroot, cucumber, lettuce, pumpkin, spinach, tofu, tomato, watercress, duck, rabbit, pork, rhubarb, banana, grapefruit, lemon and watermelon.

Yang foods are warming, dry, hard and light in colour. They are often found growing on or above ground in the presence of light, but there are exceptions such as shellfish, which are considered *yang* because of their shells. *Yang* foods include basil, chives, cinnamon, cloves, coriander, cumin, fennel, garlic, ginger, parsley, pepper, asparagus, celery, leeks, shallots, soya, chicken, lamb, mutton, apricots, cherries, chestnuts and peaches.

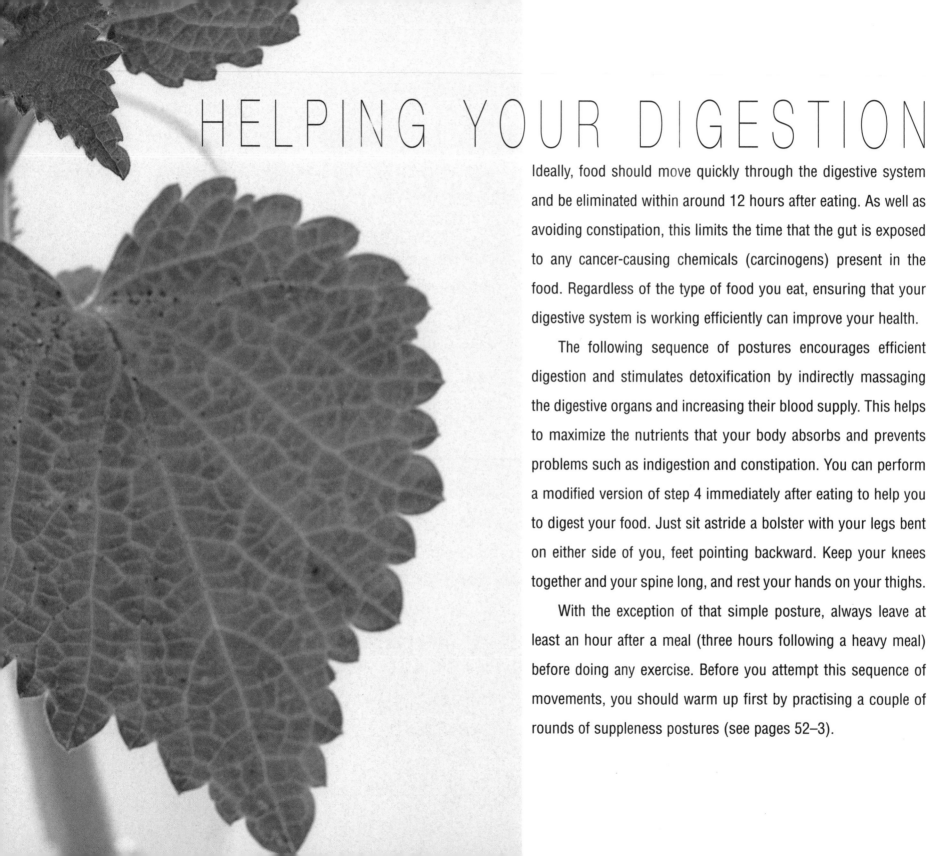

HELPING YOUR DIGESTION

Ideally, food should move quickly through the digestive system and be eliminated within around 12 hours after eating. As well as avoiding constipation, this limits the time that the gut is exposed to any cancer-causing chemicals (carcinogens) present in the food. Regardless of the type of food you eat, ensuring that your digestive system is working efficiently can improve your health.

The following sequence of postures encourages efficient digestion and stimulates detoxification by indirectly massaging the digestive organs and increasing their blood supply. This helps to maximize the nutrients that your body absorbs and prevents problems such as indigestion and constipation. You can perform a modified version of step 4 immediately after eating to help you to digest your food. Just sit astride a bolster with your legs bent on either side of you, feet pointing backward. Keep your knees together and your spine long, and rest your hands on your thighs.

With the exception of that simple posture, always leave at least an hour after a meal (three hours following a heavy meal) before doing any exercise. Before you attempt this sequence of movements, you should warm up first by practising a couple of rounds of suppleness postures (see pages 52–3).

DIGESTION SEQUENCE

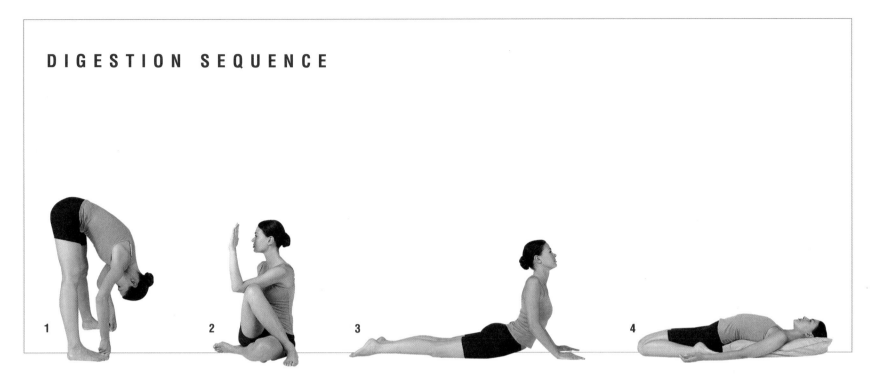

1 Stand with your feet wide apart and parallel. Put your hands on your hips, draw up your leg muscles and slowly fold forward at your hips, keeping your back straight. Grasp your ankles or toes. Concentrate on folding a little further forward on each exhalation.

2 Sit with your legs out in front, bend your left knee and let it drop out to the side. Draw your left foot under your right leg, close to your right buttock. Bend your right leg and bring your foot over your left thigh – keep right foot on the floor. Twist to the right and place your left elbow on the right knee. Put your right hand behind you for support. Turn your head to look to your right. Repeat on the other side.

3 Lie down on your front, arms bent and palms flat on the floor beneath your shoulders. Draw up your abdominal muscles, draw your shoulders back and lift your head and shoulders off the ground. Press your chest forward and up. Lift your abdomen off the floor.

4 Sit on the floor, with a large cushion just behind you. Kneel sitting back on your heels and gradually move your feet apart until you are sitting between your legs – keep your knees together. Now lean back placing your elbows on the floor for support. Gradually lower yourself on to the cushion so that your spine and head are supported. Let your arms rest loosely by your sides.

EAT MINDFULLY

STIMULATE THE SENSES

NOURISH AND DETOX

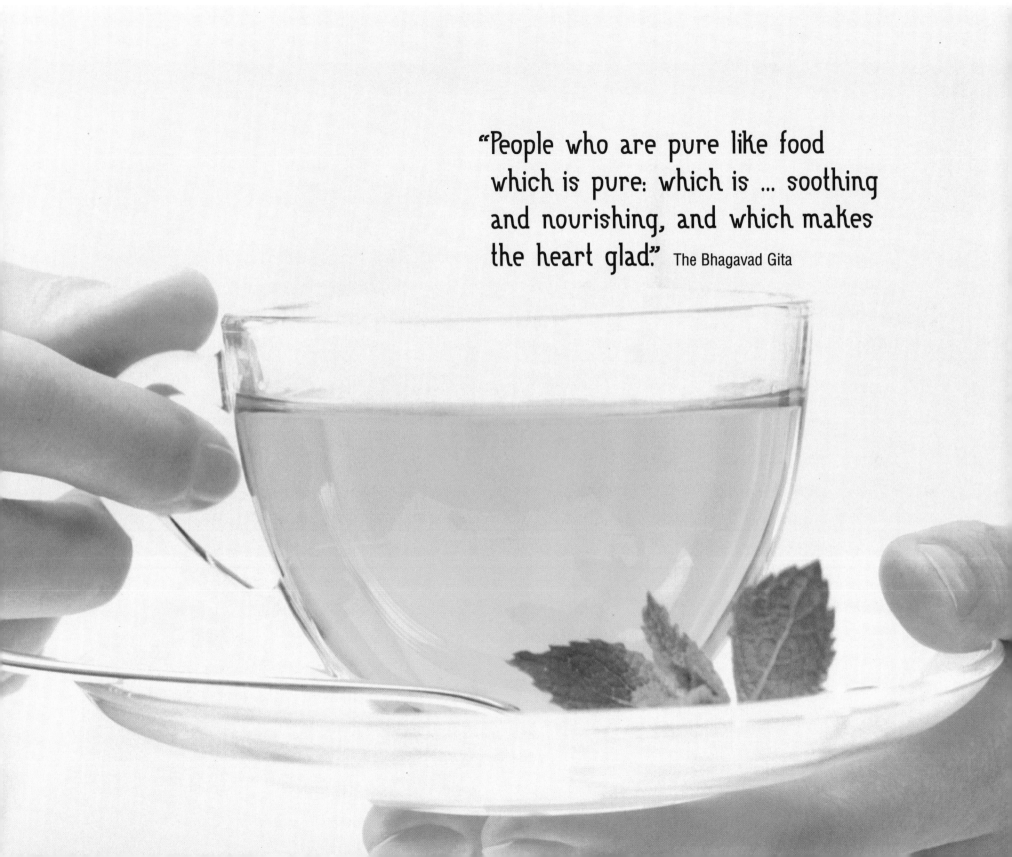

"People who are pure like food which is pure: which is ... soothing and nourishing, and which makes the heart glad." The Bhagavad Gita

THE YOGIC DIET

The yogic diet is based on the principle that we are all influenced by an interaction of three vital qualities, or *gunas*, called *sattva*, *rajas* and *tamas* – each with its own specific character. An excess of any one *guna* leads to ill health so, for optimum health, we must maintain these *gunas* in careful balance through our diet.

THE HARMONIOUS SATTVIC PERSON

The hallmark of *sattva* is harmony. The *sattvic* individual experiences a sense of purity, clarity, love and understanding in life. To work toward this state of harmony, you should increase the amount of *sattvic* foods in your diet. *Sattvic* foods are nourishing and easy to digest and are regarded as the most important components of the yogic diet. They include grains, cereals, vegetables, fruit, nuts, seeds, dairy foods, herbs, herbal teas and water.

THE FIERY RAJASIC PERSON

The distinctive feature of *rajas* is energy. Individuals who are predominantly *rajasic* in character tend to be hot, fiery and forceful, prone to stress, impatience and restlessness. People with these traits should try to decrease the influence of this *guna* by reducing the amount of *rajasic* foods they eat and increasing their intake of *sattvic* and *tamasic* foods. *Rajasic* foods are hot, bitter, sour, or salty. They include coffee, chocolate, tea, salt, fish, eggs, chilli peppers, and strong herbs and spices. You should increase your intake of *rajasic* foods only if you are predominantly *tamasic* in temperament (see below) or are suffering from temporary lethargy and fatigue and in need of an energy boost.

THE LETHARGIC TAMASIC PERSON

Tamas is characterized by stasis and inertia. *Tamasic* individuals tend to be sluggish, ponderous and prone to feelings of lethargy and depression. To become less *tamasic* you should eat more *sattvic* and *rajasic* foods and fewer *tamasic* foods.

Tamasic foods are those that are acidic, dry or old. They include mushrooms, meat, onion, garlic, fermented food, such as vinegar, reheated food and over-ripe or stale foods. Alcohol is also *tamasic*. Since *tamasic* foods are generally considered bad for you, you should only consume them when you are suffering from an excess of *rajas* – for example, if you are feeling hot, stressed and overworked.

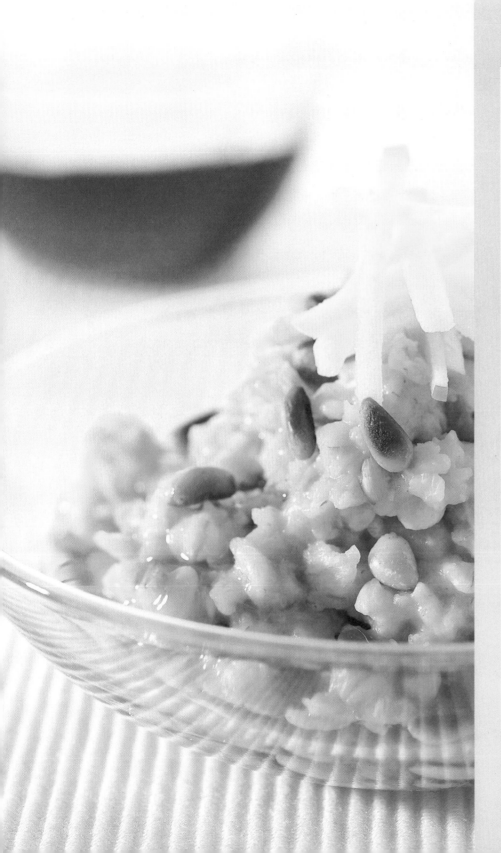

OATS WITH FRUIT AND NUTS

The following recipe makes an excellent energy-rich breakfast or snack. It contains predominantly *sattvic* foods such as nuts, grains and fruit, which are highly nutritious and aid harmony and balance.

SERVES 1

3–4 tablespoons rolled oats

1 tablespoon chopped nuts mixed with seeds
   (such as walnuts, hazelnuts, almonds, sunflower seeds)

1 tablespoon dried fruit (such as raisins or apricots)

Water

Pinch of sea salt (optional)

Soya milk

½ apple, grated

Maple syrup (optional)

Put the oats in a saucepan with the nuts, seeds and dried fruit. Add twice the volume of water and the sea salt and bring the mixture to the boil, stirring continuously. Simmer gently until the oats swell and the porridge thickens, gradually adding a little cold soya milk. Stir from time to time to prevent the porridge sticking to the pan. Serve topped with grated apple, maple syrup and soya milk to taste.

FASTING

In the East, fasting is traditionally carried out for a variety of spiritual, ritualistic, ascetic or religious reasons. In the West, fasting is becoming popular mainly for health reasons – it can improve physical and mental well-being by eliminating toxins from the body. Most of the time, our digestive system is busy breaking down food, extracting and assimilating nutrients and removing wastes. During a fast, however, the gut has a chance to rest and detoxify. As a result you feel lighter, brighter and more energized. Fasting also improves the condition of the skin and hair, aids restful sleep and boosts resistance to stress and infections, such as colds and 'flu. You may even notice an improvement in chronic health problems such as eczema, arthritis and indigestion.

WHEN TO FAST

Ideally, try to fast two to four times a year. The traditional times to fast are at the beginning of spring and autumn to energize the body for the summer and winter months ahead. Alternatively, you can fast at the beginning of each season. The following five-day dietary regime includes a 24-hour fast (on day 4) with three days of preparation and a day to readjust (you should fast for longer than a day only under the supervision of a naturopath, dietitian or nutritionist). You may lack energy during your fast, so it's sensible to choose a time when you know you won't be busy and can rest whenever you need to. Although you may not feel like doing vigorous exercise, you might find that fasting enhances your practice of yoga, t'ai chi, qigong or meditation by encouraging clear-headedness and a naturally meditative state of mind.

WORD OF WARNING

You may experience minor side effects as your body eliminates accumulated toxins, such as fatigue, headaches, irritability, bad breath, coated tongue, sugar cravings and mild palpitations. You may also feel shivery. If you suffer from more severe side effects or feel unwell, break your fast gently and consult a doctor.

Women who are pregnant or breastfeeding should never fast as it is vitally important that they maintain a high nutritional intake in order to nourish their growing baby. If you suffer from a chronic illness or are taking prescription medication, consult your doctor before fasting – never stop taking medication without seeking your doctor's advice first.

YOUR 5-DAY FAST

DAY 1: Start to prepare your body for the fast by adapting your food intake. Eliminate meat, dairy products, convenience foods, wheat products (including bread and pasta), salt, sugar, caffeinated drinks, and alcohol from your diet. Substitute these foods with rice, lentils, quinoa and buckwheat, soya products (such as soya milk) and plenty of herbal teas, water and fresh fruit and vegetables. Avoid inhaling tobacco smoke (for the entire fasting period).

DAYS 2 AND 3: Limit your diet to fruit, vegetables and plain, unsweetened yogurt. Drink plenty of fluids in the form of water, herbal teas and fruit or vegetable juices.

DAY 4: This is the day of the fast. Avoid all solid foods and throughout the day drink approximately 4 litres (7 pints) of fluid – water, herbal teas and fruit or vegetable juices. Rest when you need to. Try meditating (see page 78) – you may find you can focus more clearly or for longer than usual.

DAY 5: Your fast is now over but you should ease back into normal eating patterns gradually to give your body time to adjust. Eat lightly, concentrating on foods such as rice, yogurt and fruit and vegetables.

THE FOLLOWING WEEK: You can resume eating normally but, to consolidate the benefits of the fast, avoid salt, sugar, processed foods, alcohol, caffeine and tobacco smoke for the following week, and eat meat, particularly red meat, only in moderation.

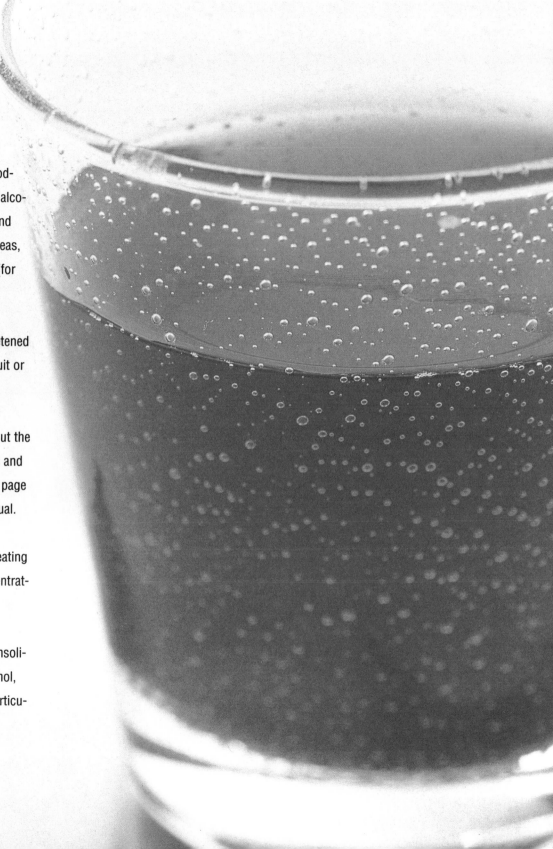

PURIFYING WATER

Medicinal teachings in the East and the West agree on the fundamental importance of water – without it, life is impossible. In Eastern terms, water is purifying – it brings life-force energy to the body and cleanses us of waste and toxins. In Western terms, water regulates all bodily processes and helps the body to extract nutrients from food. Without enough water food becomes a dry mass in the gut that the body finds difficult to break down. In the presence of sufficient water, however, the food swells and individual cells burst open to release their nutrients easily.

AVOIDING DEHYDRATION

In many ways, water is the forgotten nutrient. Although you drink enough water to survive, you may not be drinking enough fluid to keep your body adequately hydrated. You may be in a permanent state of sub-optimum hydration without realizing it. If you urinate infrequently and suffer from fatigue, lethargy, irritability, dry skin or mouth, headaches, or constipation, the chances are you're not drinking enough water. A good guide is the colour of your urine. It should be pale yellow – if it is dark amber, you need to increase your fluid intake. Ideally, you should urinate at regular intervals throughout the day – not just once or twice.

HOW MUCH TO DRINK

Aim to drink 2 litres (3$\frac{1}{2}$ pints) of water a day. Some people, especially pregnant and breastfeeding women, need even more than this. Fluid intake should be increased during hot weather, when you are taking part in vigorous exercise or if you become dehydrated as a result of vomiting or diarrhea.

Children, who tend to be more active than adults, can lose a lot of water through the skin. The average two-year-old should drink at least 500 ml (about 1 pint) a day and the average three-year-old should drink at least 750 ml (1$\frac{1}{4}$ pints).

"The removal of impurities allows the b

WHAT TO DRINK

The best way to keep the body hydrated is to drink plain water. There is much debate over the relative merits of bottled and tap water. The advantages of bottled water are that it usually provides a good source of minerals such as calcium, magnesium and potassium (check the label on the bottle) and, unlike tap water, it has not been recycled and is free from contaminants.

The advantages of tap water are that it is available cheaply and in abundance, it doesn't have to be kept refrigerated and there is no cost to the environment in terms of the disposal of plastic bottles. If you are concerned about tap water quality, speak to your local water company or try using a water filter.

If you find it unpalatable to drink plain water, you can enhance the taste using natural flavourings such as root ginger, lemon or lime juice, fresh mint leaves or a dash of elderflower cordial. Alternatively, you can mix water with fruit juice or make herbal tea. Try to limit drinks that contain caffeine as these reduce fluid levels in the body by increasing the rate of urination.

HOW TO DRINK MORE

Thirst is a useful reminder to drink, but it is not a very accurate indicator of your body's true fluid levels. By the time you feel thirsty your body cells and tissues are already in serious need of water. A better approach is to drink before you feel thirsty – this way you keep your body topped up with fluid all the time.

One way to do this is to drink little and often throughout the day – having a small bottle beside you that you can keep filling up acts as a good reminder. Alternatively, you can start the day by consuming a large amount of water on an empty stomach (up to 1 litre/1³/₄ pint, if possible). It is preferable to drink water on an empty stomach because drinking on a full stomach can dilute your digestive juices and may impede your ability to digest food.

y to function more efficiently." Yoga Sutras Upanishad

HEALTH-GIVING TEA

In the West, the word "tea" usually makes us think of a hot drink made from black leaves. In fact, there are thousands of types of tea leaf, all derived from the evergreen *Camellia sinensis*. Variations in flavour, aroma and colour depend on the growing conditions for the plant and the methods of picking, processing, storing and packaging practised in different tea-growing regions.

Tea contains caffeine, a chemical stimulant more often associated with coffee. This chemical not only stimulates the nervous system, making us feel jittery, and interferes with sleep quality, but it also acts as a diuretic and so reduces fluid levels in the body. Yet tea also enhances health because of substances called polyphenols (or flavonoids) in its leaves. Polyphenols have antioxidant properties, which means they mop up harmful substances known as free radicals that are produced naturally by the body and also generated by tobacco smoke and pollution. Polyphenols help to prevent degenerative diseases, such as cancer, heart disease and premature ageing, and they also lower levels of "bad" cholesterol.

The best way to mitigate the effects of caffeine and to benefit from antioxidant polyphenols is to drink tea in moderation (one or two cups a day), avoid caffeinated drinks after mid-afternoon (as they may interfere with sleep) and switch to less processed types of tea, such as green tea. Green tea has been used medicinally in the East for centuries. Its leaves are steamed or roasted soon after picking, which kills the oxidizing enzymes that would otherwise cause the chemical reactions responsible for the darker colour and stronger flavour of black-leaf tea. As a result, green tea retains high levels of polyphenols, which may partly explain Japan's low rate of heart disease. It is also worthwhile experimenting with other types of tea. Try Assam (see recipe, right), oolong or lapsang souchong teas, for example.

AID TO CONTEMPLATION

You can also drink tea as a contemplative act. In Japan, many people perform an elaborate ritual, derived from Zen Buddhism, known as a tea ceremony (*chanoyu*). During this ceremony, host and guests follow a highly formalized system of gestures and actions designed to focus the minds of participants. This frees them to become absorbed in the moment and meditate as they drink. Tea is drunk from a small bowl – itself a spiritual symbol.

INDIAN CHAI TEA

This tea is full of warming aromatic spices that have various health benefits. Chai tea is widely drunk in northern India and has a delicious and comforting incense smell.

1 tablespoon ginger powder
2 teaspoons cardamom seeds, ground
4 cloves, ground
1 teaspoon black peppercorns, ground
1 teaspoon cinnamon powder
1 teaspoon star anise, ground (optional)
4 teaspoons Assam tea
1 litre/1¾ pints water
Milk and honey to taste

Mix all the spices together and store in a well-sealed jar. To make 4 cups of tea, boil 1 teaspoon of the spice mixture together with the Assam tea and water. Simmer on a low heat for 5 minutes. Add milk to taste and bring back to the boil. Strain into cups and add honey to taste. Serve hot.

THE JOY OF JUICING

Drinking fruit and vegetable juices is a delicious way to pack lots of extra vitamins and minerals into your diet. Western dietary guidelines advocate eating at least five portions of fruit and vegetables every day – and drinking just one freshly squeezed mixed juice recipe a day can account for up to half of your recommended intake. From an Eastern perspective, juices are full of life-force energy, they cleanse the body and help to prevent disease.

FRESHLY MADE AND FUN TO DRINK

The best way to benefit from the health-giving properties of juices is to make them freshly at home. Commercially prepared juices often have sugar, flavourings or preservatives added. If you do drink shop-bought juices, whenever possible choose brands that are organically produced and unsweetened.

To juice fruit and vegetables at home you need a few basic pieces of equipment including a squeezer for extracting the juice from citrus fruit (this doesn't have to be an elaborate device – an old-fashioned lemon squeezer is fine) and an electric juicer for extracting the juice from other types of fruit and vegetable, such as carrots and apples (electric juicers often contain an attachment for citrus fruit). A blender is also useful for making smoothies and liquidizing whole soft fruits such as blueberries, raspberries, strawberries or bananas.

Make the juice from the freshest fruit and vegetables you can buy or, if you can, harvest your own produce. Always wash fruit and vegetables thoroughly and discard produce that is damaged or decaying. Freshly squeezed juice doesn't keep for long and quickly becomes discoloured when in contact with the air. For this reason, it's best to make juice in small quantities and drink it immediately. Alternatively, a small amount of fresh lemon juice added to a juice can preserve it for a short time.

MIX YOUR OWN JUICY COMBINATIONS

Why not make your own juice cocktails? You can be as inventive as you like – combine the juices of your favourite fruit and vegetables and see what works best. Carrot and apple juice is a refreshing combination; so is apple and mango or pineapple and grapefruit. "Juicy" vegetables such as tomatoes and cucumber are popular choices, but you can also try other vegetables such as beetroot, celery, onion, lettuce, watercress and spinach.

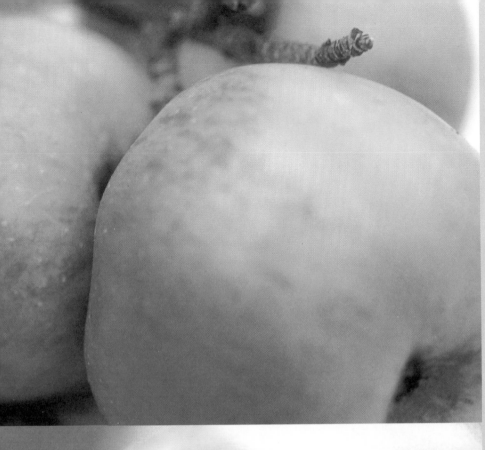

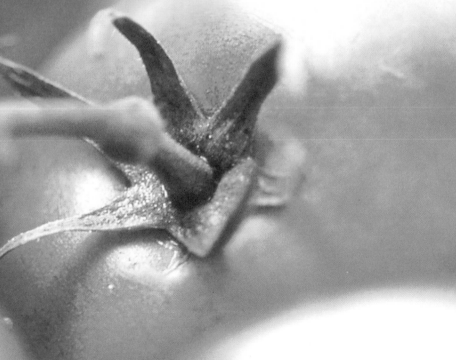

The following recipes are packed with nutrients. Dawn Chorus is a great wake-up call to the body at breakfast time. Party Popper is a delicious non-alcoholic cocktail and can also be served as an appetizer.

DAWN CHORUS

4 apples, peeled and cored

2 pears, peeled and cored

½ lemon, squeezed

1 teaspoon maple syrup

Juice the apples and pears. Add the lemon juice and maple syrup. Mix well and serve in a tall glass.

PARTY POPPER

3 sticks celery

3 medium tomatoes

½ cucumber

½ lime, squeezed

Dash of Worcestershire sauce

Salt and pepper to taste

Wash and then juice the celery, tomatoes and cucumber. Add the lime juice and Worcestershire sauce. Season, if liked, mix well and serve.

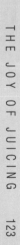

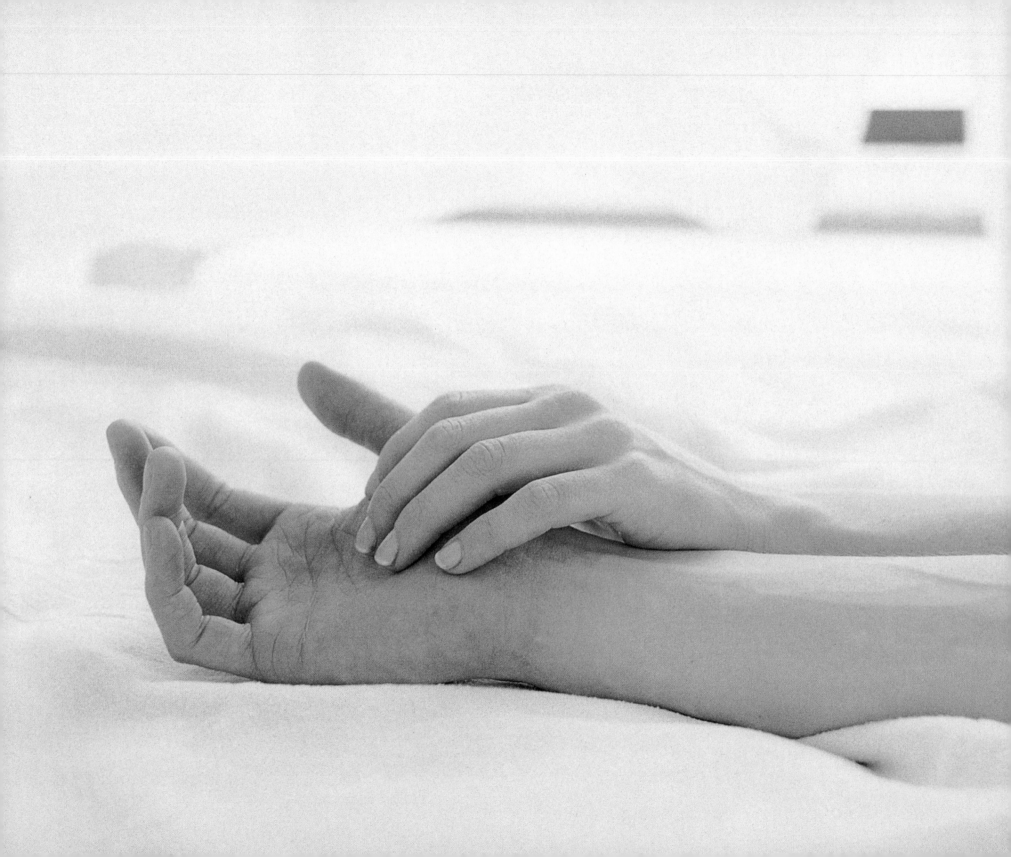

LOVING

The ability to love others in an open-hearted and uncritical way not only enhances your own life and the lives of those around you, but also opens the gateway to your emotional and spiritual development. In Buddhism, the art of loving yourself and other people compassionately is one of the first and most basic teachings.

This chapter looks at how to surrender selfish and possessive approaches to relationships and replace them with feelings of warmth, empathy and generosity. The spiritual approach of Buddhism is combined with techniques, such as Indian head massage, that can greatly increase intimacy through the power of touch.

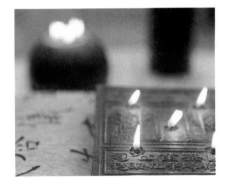

LOVING KINDNESS

As we grow older we tend to lose the ability to relate to others in the open-hearted and unconditional way we did as children. We may become reserved about showing love and affection, and more judgmental in our relationships or cynical about human nature in general. Gradually, many of our interactions with others become characterized by negative feelings. One of the central tenets of Buddhism is the complete and selfless love of others. This not only offers a route to spiritual awakening but can also greatly improve your quality of life and that of those around you.

Buddhist teachers advocate meditation as a way of opening your heart and experiencing more love and compassion. They recommend a meditation technique known as *metta bhavana* (*metta* means "love" and *bhavana* means "development").

PRACTISING *METTA BHAVANA*

To prepare for *metta bhavana*, sit on the floor in a cross-legged or other meditative position (see pages 80–1) and close your eyes. Breathe evenly and steadily through your nose and try to focus on the feelings of love that lie dormant within you. To do this, cast your mind back to a time when you felt really loved. You might recall the unconditional love that your parents or other adults showed you as a child, or a particular occasion when you felt moved by a friend's kindness and generosity. Concentrate on what it felt like to be loved. Try to love and accept yourself as completely and unconditionally as that – it will enable you to cultivate and extend love to others. At first, tapping into feelings of love, particularly self-love, can be difficult and may make you feel uncomfortable. Keep trying – it will become easier with time.

The next stage is to direct these feelings toward others. Your aim is to break down boundaries so that, ultimately, you are able to extend feelings of love and compassion to everyone around you – not just those whom you care for already.

Try to direct feelings of love to the following types of people in this order: a highly esteemed or respected person, such as a teacher, colleague or spiritual leader; a close friend or relative; a neutral person whom you encounter on a daily basis but do not know very well, such as a person who serves you in a shop; a hostile person with whom you are currently having problems. You'll find this stage of your meditation much easier if you use techniques such as visualization (see page 158). As you think of

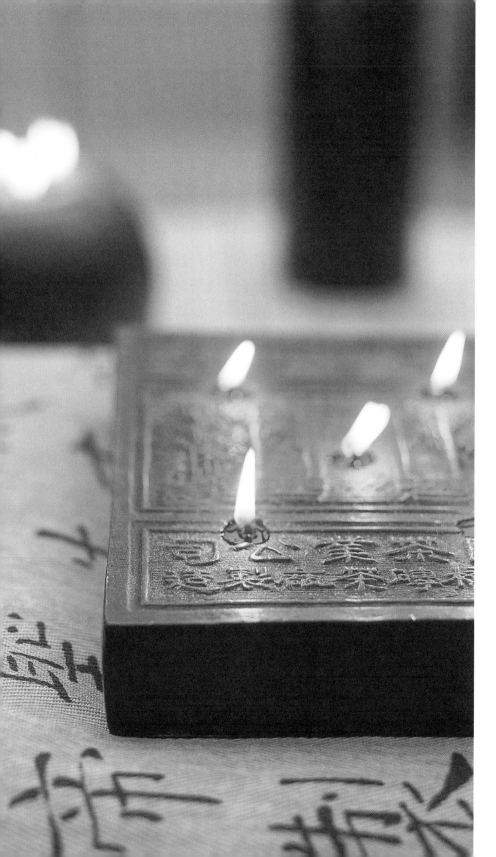

someone, imagine them standing in front of you smiling and looking happy. You can send them loving thoughts such as "may you be free from harm and suffering" or "may you be safe and happy". You may find it helpful to repeat the words "loving kindness" silently as a mantra as you think about your chosen person.

If you find this difficult, especially toward those in the latter part of the list, remind yourself that everyone is fundamentally the same: we all have the same feelings, the same desires for happiness and contentment, and the same fears of pain and suffering. Try to feel empathy for fellow human beings and to replace old feelings of resentment, bitterness or anger with compassion.

When you feel you have succeeded in directing love to particular people you can try the final stage of this loving kindness meditation which involves extending love indiscriminately to people and cultures all over the world. Try to feel that you can radiate love without reservations or boundaries. Once you reach this stage, you should feel you are able to love freely and unconditionally. Practise these loving feelings not just in meditation, but in your day-to-day life so that you greet everyone around you with warmth, openness, compassion and empathy.

ENHANCING INTIMACY

Intimacy is often lost in many modern relationships because couples are too busy or tired to touch. This can lead to feelings of being disconnected from one another. The simple act of doing exercises together can help to bring back the loving connection. The following stretches offer a wonderful way to spend quality time together and also enhance intimacy between you. In this sequence you need to depend on your partner to give you exactly the right amount of support at the right time – this provides a valuable lesson in communication. Prepare by warming up with a few rounds of the suppleness sequence on page 52. Take turns in the supporting role. Experiment by giving different amounts of support and ask each other what you find most helpful.

A good way to "tune in" with your partner while doing these stretches (and at other times, too) is to synchronize breathing. Spend a few minutes sitting quietly back to back. Breathe deeply through your nose and concentrate on the movement of your partner's back expanding and contracting against yours with each breath. Keep breathing deeply, and gradually bring your breathing into line with your partner's – this will help to ground and connect you. Try to maintain this synchrony throughout the sequence.

LOVING STRETCHES

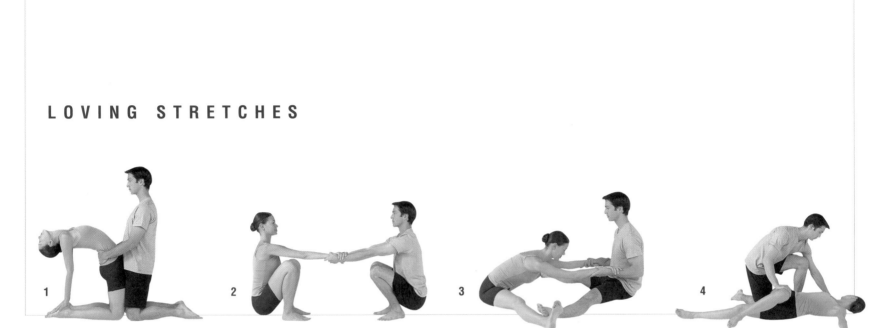

1 Kneel up with your thighs at right angles to your calves and your knees close together and parallel. Your partner kneels in front of you and puts his hands behind your back for support. Now push your chest up and lean into a backbend. Bring your hands down to hold your heels and let your head drop gently back. Let your partner's support help you to increase the backbend.

2 Stand facing your partner and grasp each other's wrists. Slowly straighten your arms in front of you so that you are both leaning back. Using each other as a counterweight, bend your knees and come slowly down into a deep squat. Return to standing in the same way.

3 Sit facing each other. Stretch your legs out to the sides as far as is comfortable. Your partner places his feet on your inner ankles. Grasp each other's wrists. As you exhale, your partner gently pulls you toward him. Keep your knees and toes pointing upward.

4 Lie on your back and bring your right knee up to your chest. Let it drop to the left side. Now turn your head to face right. Your partner kneels by your right side and assists the stretch by placing his left hand on your right shoulder and his right hand on your right knee and gently pushes down. Repeat the stretch on the other side. Swap roles and end with a sitting embrace (shown beneath this page).

LOVE UNCRITICALLY

EMBRACE INTIMACY

DEVELOP SPIRITUALLY

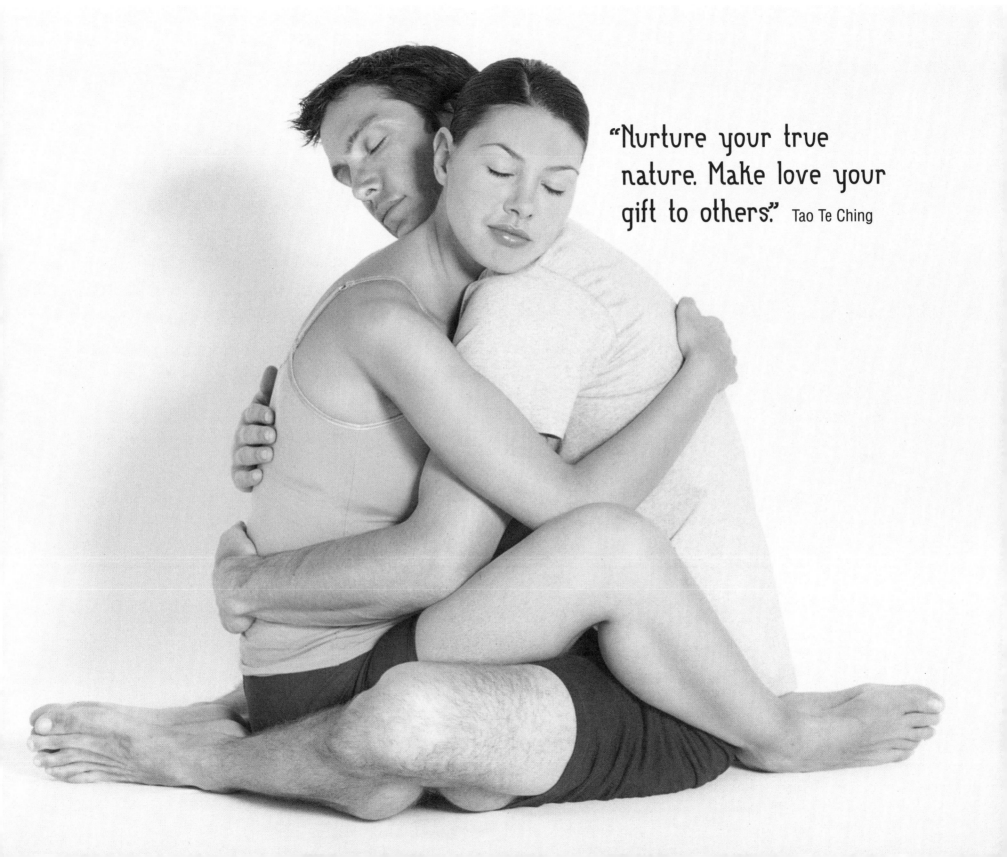

"Nurture your true nature. Make love your gift to others." Tao Te Ching

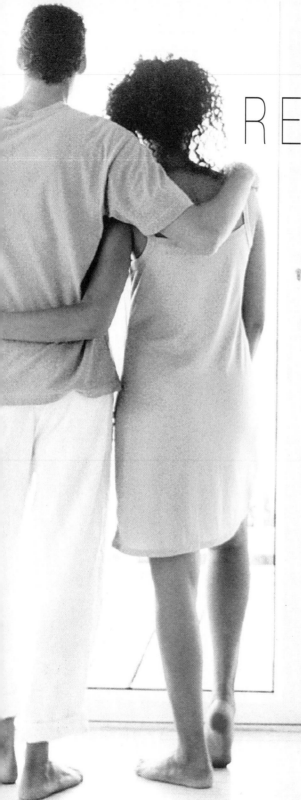

RELEASING ATTACHMENT

Good relationships make you feel loved, wanted and cared for. They give you courage and confidence and reassure you that you are not alone. They even recreate the warm climate of childhood when – hopefully – you felt safe and protected. Unfortunately, these positive aspects of relationships can be combined with negative aspects. Many relationships falter because of the fear that we'll lose our partners. Perhaps they'll grow bored, meet someone else or simply fall out of love with us.

The fear of abandonment can make us defensive and reluctant to reveal our emotions, preventing an honest and open connection between two people; it can make us needy, dependent and possessive; it can force us into playing games to test our partner's commitment; and it can make us aggressive, suspicious or violent, as we strive for more control.

Such attempts to cling on to relationships are counterproductive – instead of bringing the happiness and contentment we crave, they mire us in fear and discontentment. According to Buddhist philosophy, the way out of this fear trap is not to seek more control within the relationship but rather to seek less: to stop striving so hard and simply let go. This is the principle of non-grasping or non-attachment. In the words of Sogyal Rinpoche, author of *The Tibetan Book of Living and Dying*: "Although we have been made to believe that if we let go we will end up with nothing, life itself reveals again and again the opposite: that letting go is the path to happiness".

LOOSEN YOUR GRIP

In Buddhism, love is defined by kindness, compassion and empathy. Attachment is characterized by insecurity, possessiveness and pride. Letting go of attachment necessitates a leap in the way that we perceive relationships – it involves accepting the possibility of impermanence. Buddhists compare grasping at love to grasping at life – both are futile because love and life are, by nature, ungraspable. The route to happiness is to relax your grip.

Letting go of attachment doesn't mean becoming detached, cold or distant. Instead, your relationships should become more warm and loving because you will be devoting your energy to ensuring your partner's happiness and less energy trying to bend the relationship to fit your own needs. Whenever you make a demand or have an argument, ask yourself what your motivation

is: love and compassion or fear and insecurity? Learn to distinguish between the childish voice of your ego (see page 64) and the voice of your true self, which allows you and those around you the freedom to express your individual wishes and desires, without fearing that this will threaten the relationship.

PRACTISE LETTING GO

Start by carrying out the loving kindness meditation on page 126. Then perform the following visualization exercise. Imagine you have a coin in your hand that represents a relationship you are afraid of losing. You are holding the coin tightly in your fist with your palm turned downward – if you open your hand the coin will drop to the floor so you must keep your fist closed as tightly as possible. Now imagine the opposite scenario. You turn your fist over so that your fingers face upward and uncurl your fingers one by one until your hand is outstretched. Although the coin is surrounded by boundless space it continues to lie securely in your palm. Imagine the feeling of calm that this brings. Try to look at your partner in the same light – think how supporting, sharing and nurturing him or her will keep them secure in your love.

OVERCOMING PROBLEMS

All relationships face difficulties from time to time. But many people respond to disputes by digging themselves into defensive positions and automatically blaming the other person. A better approach, and one that's in line with the Buddhist principle of "loving kindness", is to accept problems with equanimity and attempt to understand the reasons that lie behind them. When you avoid apportioning blame you acknowledge that the causes of every problem are complex and not the fault of any one person.

The next time you find yourself in dispute with your partner, ask yourself the following questions. Are you angry because you feel hurt? If so, why not say so openly and explain why? Do you ever behave in a similar way and, if so, why? If your partner is acting out of unhappiness, what is the reason? Instead of reacting to a situation with anger and resentment, aim to challenge your habitual responses and show tolerance and understanding. This approach helps build a deeper sense of connection with your partner so that problems are less likely to occur in future.

Arguments can develop into situations where people become so dogmatic they may even end up defending a view they don't hold. Instead of adopting an entrenched position, try to take an impartial overview that allows you to be more understanding and forgiving. The following exercises will help you to empathize with your partner and see things from their perspective. The next time things get heated, agree to break off and do this exercise. Imagine you are sitting with your partner and cast your mind back to a time when the relationship was harmonious and you could speak freely. Imagine this is still the case. Visualize your partner with an open expression being receptive to what you say. Now explain the problem non-judgmentally. Imagine saying how angry, hurt or upset you've been feeling. Visualize letting go of all your defences and speaking openly.

To take this exercise a stage further, you could write an imaginary dialogue. Put down what you have just said and then write down what your partner would say to you in this new climate of understanding. Let him or her explain their side of the problem. Keep writing both sides of the dialogue until you feel everything has been said. When you resume, give the dialogue to each other to read. The exercise should help you to open a new, more sensitive dialogue with the person in real life. You may then be able to sort out future problems with greater understanding.

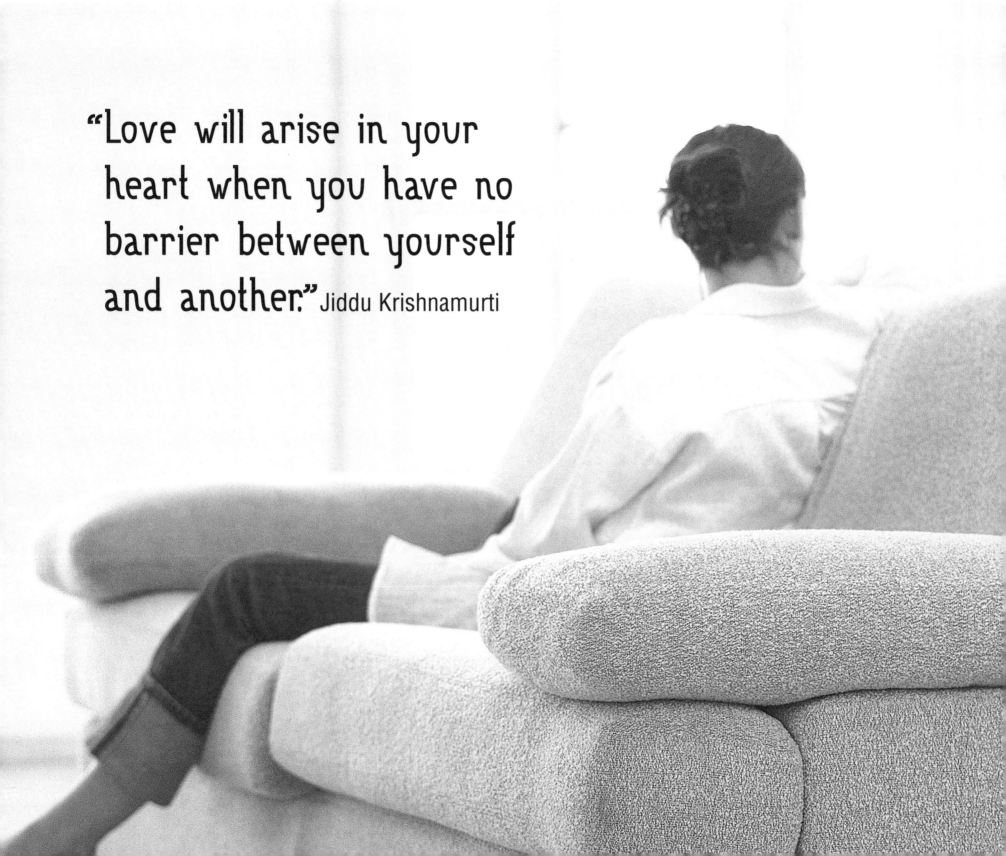

"Love will arise in your heart when you have no barrier between yourself and another." Jiddu Krishnamurti

Head massage has a long tradition in India. Parents massage their children's hair to encourage thick and lustrous growth, and barbers offer head massage as a service to clients. You can even get a head massage on beaches and street corners. The benefits are profound – as well as being relaxing and sensual, head massage brings feelings of peace, reassurance and comfort. The caring, soothing touch of head massage strengthens relationships by enhancing the sense of sharing and trust between partners. Head massage also provides the perfect antidote to stress at the end of a hectic, tension-filled day and helps create a mood of relaxation and intimacy that often leads to lovemaking.

It is standard practice to use scented oils such as coconut, sesame, mustard or almond. The oils enable the hands to flow over the scalp and the fragrances of the individual oils have their own unique properties. The hair also benefits from a root-to-tip conditioning treatment. You can buy oils ready-made or make your own by adding a few drops of essential oil (sandalwood, jasmine or cinnamon are popular) to a base oil such as sunflower oil.

There are no strict rules about how to give a head massage. In India, each family uses its own special techniques, which are passed down from one generation to the next. The following sequence gives a wonderfully sensual head massage. You can adapt the strokes to your own needs or make up your own. Ask your partner what feels good and be guided by him or her. If you wish, you can incorporate the neck and shoulders into your massage, or use head massage as a finale to a full body massage.

Make sure your massage partner is sitting comfortably in an aligned position (see page 44) with eyes shut. Keep one hand in contact with his or her head at all times and make your strokes smooth and flowing so that it's hard to tell where one stroke ends and the next begins. Breathe slowly and deeply – your partner will pick up on this and slow their own breathing accordingly.

SENSUAL HEAD MASSAGE

Rub some oil into your palms and stroke your hands through your partner's hair using long, sweeping movements from the crown of the head to the back of the scalp. Add more oil to your palms until you have spread oil evenly through the hair. Support your partner's forehead with one hand and use the heel of the other to apply pressure to the base of the skull (shown right). Rub

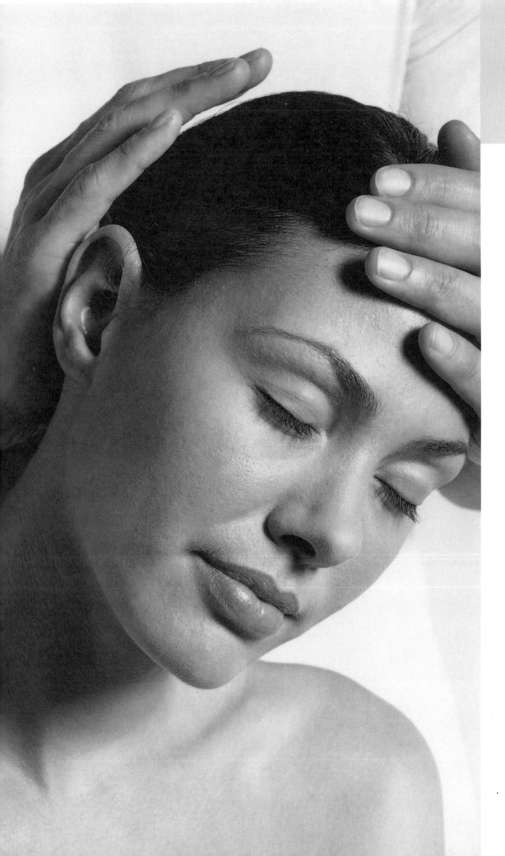

lightly up and down with the heel of your hand all across the back of the head. Now, starting at the top of the head, gather sections of hair in both your fists and make gentle tugging movements. Cover the whole head in this way.

Spread your fingers wide and use the pads of your fingers and thumbs to make small circular movements all over the head, feeling the scalp moving under your hands. Holding your fingers in the same position, tap lightly all over the head, keeping your fingers flexible and your movements quick and light.

Rest the heels of your hands on either side of your partner's head just above the ears with your fingertips resting on top of the head. Apply pressure and then gently push the scalp up. Repeat with the heels of your hands just in front of the ears.

Place the palms of your hands over the temples with fingers outstretched. Using gentle pressure, move your palms in big, slow circles over the temples. Repeat this action over the ears using very gentle pressure. To finish, rest your hands on top of your partner's head with fingers pointing away from you and gently stroke the hair downward, using alternate hands. Now swap roles so each of you enjoys the delights of a partner's touch.

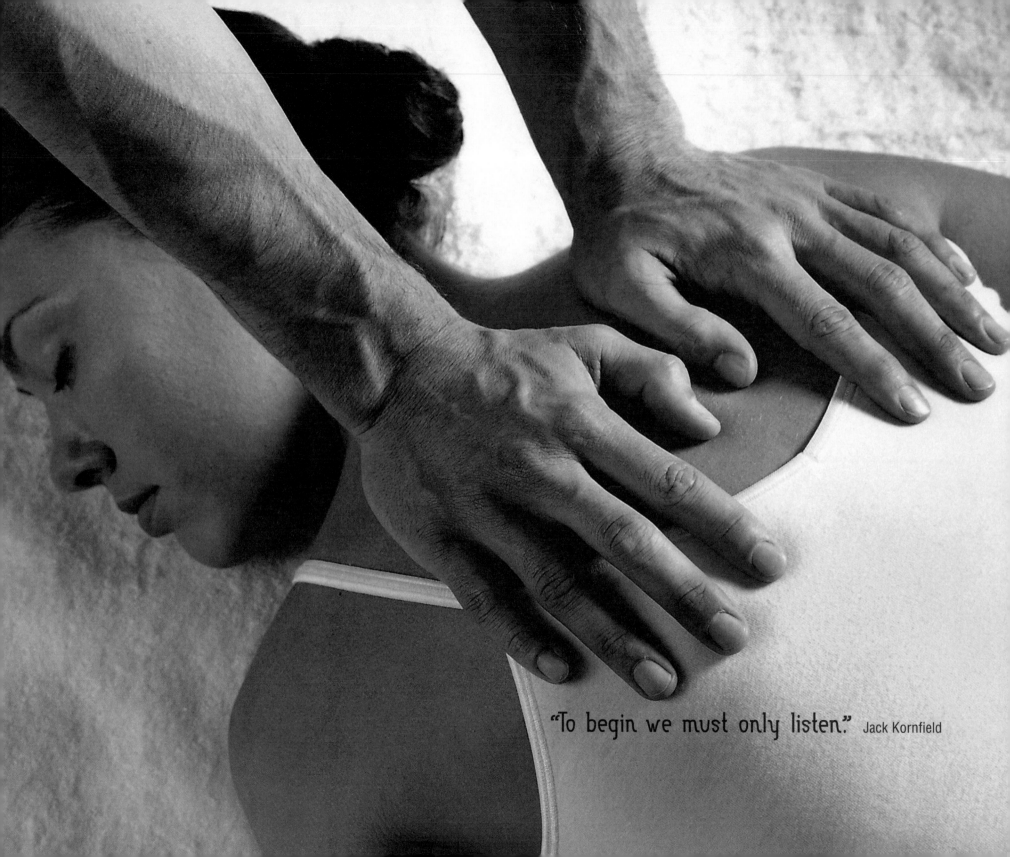

"To begin we must only listen." Jack Kornfield

CONTACT AND FOCUS

A shiatsu back massage allows you to enjoy close contact with your partner and also enhances feelings of trust and intimacy. Shiatsu is an ancient Japanese therapy that aims to balance the flow of *ki* energy (equivalent to *qi* or *chi*) along channels in the body. If you and your partner are facing a big decision, such as whether or not to get married, have a baby, or move house, the following massage can help. It helps to integrate the brain and nervous system, so alleviating feelings of anxiety, restlessness, confusion and indecision. To ensure that you both benefit fully from the massage, take the telephone off the hook and find a quiet room where you will be undisturbed. This is "you" time, when you must concentrate fully on one another – the best mutual decisions are made when you are both fully focused and relaxed.

SHIATSU BACK MASSAGE

This massage uses a simple palm-pressure technique in which you place your hands on your partner's body and slowly bring your body weight to bear down through your hands. Wear loose clothing that allows you to move freely. Your partner can be dressed or undressed to receive the massage. He or she should be lying face down on the floor, comfortably supported on a firm surface, such as futon mattress, or several layers of blankets.

Kneel by your partner's side and place your palms on either side of his or her waist. Transfer some of your body weight to your hands. Slowly walk your hands back toward your partner's sacrum (the part of the spine between the hip bones) applying firm pressure at each step. Now get astride your partner and link fingers. Rest your linked hands on your partner's sacrum and press down firmly using your body weight.

Move to your partner's head, keeping one hand on his or her back for reassurance as you do so. Kneel and place your hands between his or her shoulderblades. Press down firmly. Now place your hands on either side of the spine (shown opposite) and walk your palms down the length of his or her back. Lean forward to keep your body weight centred over your palms.

Take turns to perform the massage so that you both enjoy the benefits. As you perform the massage, talk over the problem you must decide on. The massage will help you and your partner to feel relaxed and focused, more in tune with one another, so making it easier to arrive at a decision you can both agree on.

SEX AND SPIRITUALITY

In the West, we have come to expect a great deal from sex. Magazines, books, films, television and advertisements lead us to believe that sexual intimacy should fulfil all our needs for love, passion, excitement and romance. It is as though good sex equals happiness, contentment and success, and bad sex – or no sex – equals misery, discontentment and personal failure.

In contrast, the approach of some Eastern disciplines is far less goal-oriented. For example, the Indian art of Tantrism (and the Chinese art of Taoism) considers sex to be a valuable union between two equal but opposing masculine and feminine energy forces. In Tantrism, these forces are known as *Shiva* and *Shakti* (in Taoism they are called *yin* and *yang*). Sexual union is perceived as a way of achieving a balance of energies and, as such, is considered vital to both physical and spiritual health.

THE TANTRIC APPROACH TO SEX

Tantrism is a branch of yoga that derives from a set of scriptures known as the *Tantras*, some of which are concerned with erotic instruction. According to Tantrism, sex offers a valuable way of harnessing energy to achieve a state of higher consciousness or enlightenment. By prolonging intercourse, avoiding orgasm and ejaculation and controlling the breath, practitioners transform sex into a meditative act that aids spiritual development.

Although not all Westerners may choose to seek spiritual enlightenment through sex, Tantrism can still provide a valuable lesson in intimacy, sensuality and bonding. For many couples, the only purpose of sex is to achieve an orgasm. Not only can this put performance pressure on both men and women and make partners feel inadequate if they don't climax, it also means that orgasm represents an abrupt full stop to sensual pleasure.

Tantrism advocates a technique known as "riding the edge of the wave" which enables couples to make love for several hours before – or without – climaxing. Some people find that removing the "necessity" to have an orgasm makes sex more enjoyable and enhances an awareness of the bond with their partner.

HOW TO RIDE THE WAVE

The aim of "riding the wave" is to achieve a meditative state during sex. Ideally, this should be learned from an expert but it's possible to practise your own version using the following techniques.

First, prepare for sex with a slow and sensual build-up. Feed each other with exotic foods and take turns to wash and then massage each other with scented oils. This helps to establish a mood of complete intimacy and relaxation.

Sit facing each other cross-legged on the floor and quietly concentrate on your breathing. After a few moments, place your right hands lightly on each other's chest, just over the heart. Feel the warmth of your partner's skin. Begin to synchronize your breathing – concentrate on the rise and fall of inhalation and exhalation. Become aware of each other's heartbeat through the palm of your hands. Breathe slowly into your abdomen, gaze deeply into each other's eyes and focus your thoughts exclusively on each other. Imagine your loving feelings pouring through your hand into your partner, and their love pouring into you.

When you are ready to make love, a recommended position is one in which the man stays sitting cross-legged on the floor and the woman sits on top of him with her legs around his waist. As this is a fairly static position, it enables you to keep looking deep into each other's eyes and meditating upon one another.

To maintain erotic intensity, the woman can contract her vaginal muscles around the man's penis. If the man becomes too aroused he can prevent himself ejaculating by concentrating on his breathing and lengthening his exhalation (this is a good delaying tactic for any type of sex). If the man becomes tired, he can lie on his back while the woman sits astride him with her hands on his chest. Bear in mind that your ultimate goal is not to reach orgasm but to enjoy a sense of sensuality, deep bonding and union with your partner.

"As long as there is the desire to gain...
there is anxiety, sorrow and fear." Jiddu Krishnamurti

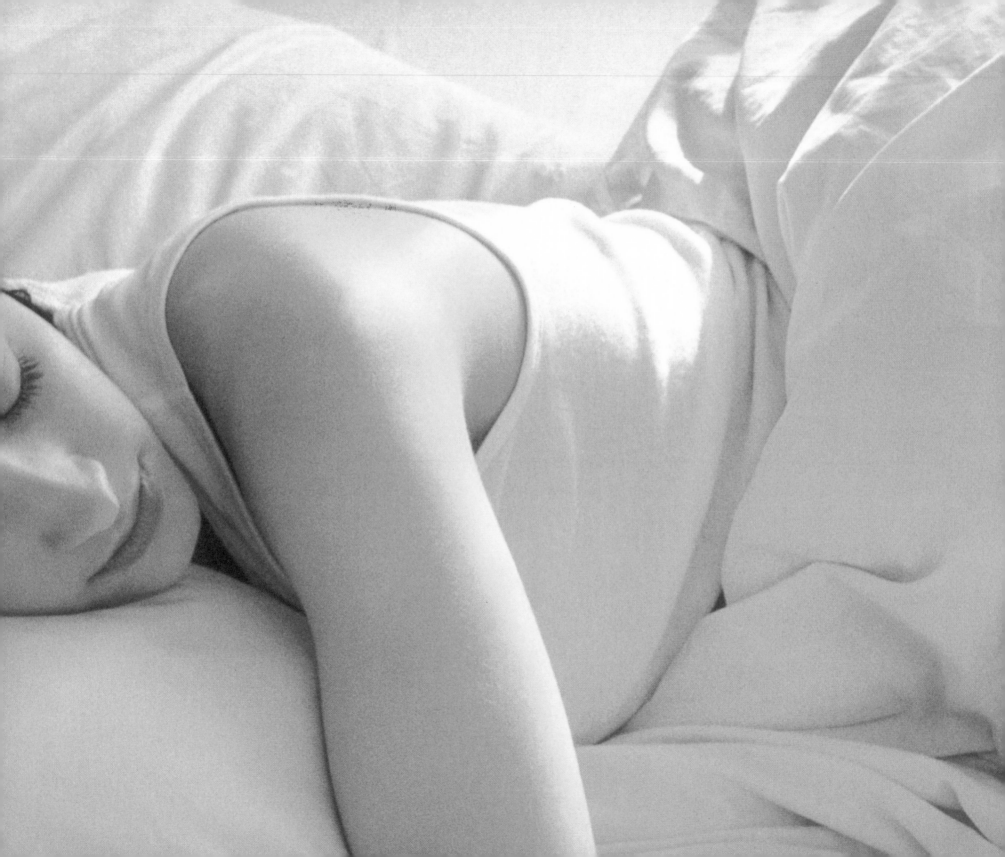

SLEEPING

The key to a good night's rest is complete physical and mental relaxation in the

wind-down period before you go to bed. Muscles all over the body can harbour

tension from long periods spent sitting or standing at work and the mind is

frequently busy processing the day's events or mulling over problems.

   This chapter shows you how to rid yourself of stress, tension and anxiety and

prepare for sleep using a wide range of therapies and techniques, from yoga

breathing and visualization to stretching sequences and feng shui. After enjoying

a good night's rest you will wake feeling refreshed and ready to face the new day.

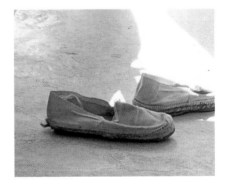

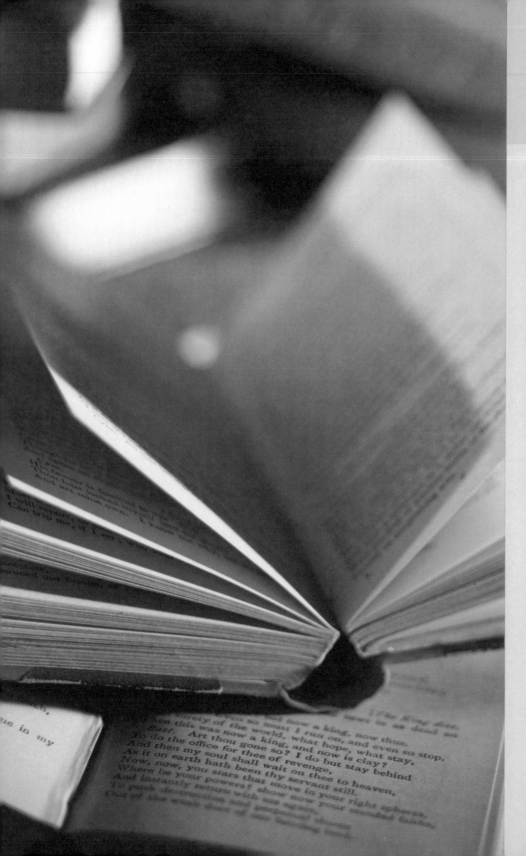

WINDING DOWN

It is important to allow yourself a little time at the end of the day to wind down and relax, ready for bed. If you try to go to sleep immediately after working or watching television, you'll find that your mind is crammed with thoughts and your body is still tense. You should also avoid drinking coffee or doing vigorous exercise too late in the evening, as this can stimulate your mind and body. Instead, set aside an hour or so of "quiet time" that you can devote to restful activities such as reading, yoga or meditation. Both of the following calming techniques: progressive muscle relaxation and Brahmari breath are great ways of winding down.

RELAX YOUR MUSCLES

Progressive muscle relaxation is a thorough and systematic way of releasing tension from your body. Simply lie down on your back in the corpse pose (see page 93), take a few moments to relax and then flex your feet and clench your toes – try to make your feet as tense as possible. After about five seconds, let your feet relax and become completely floppy and feel the tension drain away from them. Tell yourself that your feet feel warm and heavy, and enjoy the sensation that this creates. Try to be aware of the opposite sensations that tension and relaxation produce – this awareness is the key to learning to relax at will. For example, if you notice a melting or tingling sensation in your feet as they relax, remember this sensation to target tension spots later on.

Now, repeat this tensing and relaxing process with your calves and work your way up your body, concentrating on each set of muscles in turn: thighs, buttocks, pelvic floor muscles, abdomen, lower back, chest, upper back, hands (make them into fists), forearms, upper arms, shoulders and throat. When you reach your face, open your mouth wide and stick your tongue out as far as it will go. Then close your mouth, screw your eyes up and make your forehead into a deep frown. Now relax your entire face and scalp. Feel your head fully supported by the floor.

By this stage, all the major muscle groups have been tensed and relaxed and you should now feel that your body is heavy, and resting with its full weight on the floor. Spend as long as you like immersed in this relaxed state. Imagine that your mind is like a spotlight that roams up and down your body looking for areas of tension. If and when it detects a tense spot, remember how it felt to let go of tension and try to experience this feeling again.

BREATHE YOURSELF TO SLEEP

A yoga breathing exercise called Brahmari breath (also known as humming bee breath – "Brahmari" means "bee") is a great way to induce a light meditative state before you go to sleep. As you exhale, you make a sound like a bee and this helps you feel calm and relaxed. Brahmari breath naturally helps you to lengthen your exhalation. This is therapeutic because exhalation is believed to have a tranquillizing effect on the mind. Brahmari breath also releases tension in the muscles of the neck, throat, upper back and shoulders that can build up during the day.

Sit cross-legged on the floor and block your ears with your fingers. Inhale and exhale a few times, concentrating on the sound of your breathing. Notice how your breath sounds different with the ears closed – this sound is calming in itself. Now make a humming sound on your next exhalation. Play around with the pitch and volume until you make a soothing hum. Keep making the sound as you exhale until you feel that your lungs are almost empty. Then inhale. Repeat this ten times.

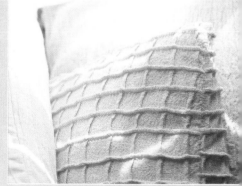

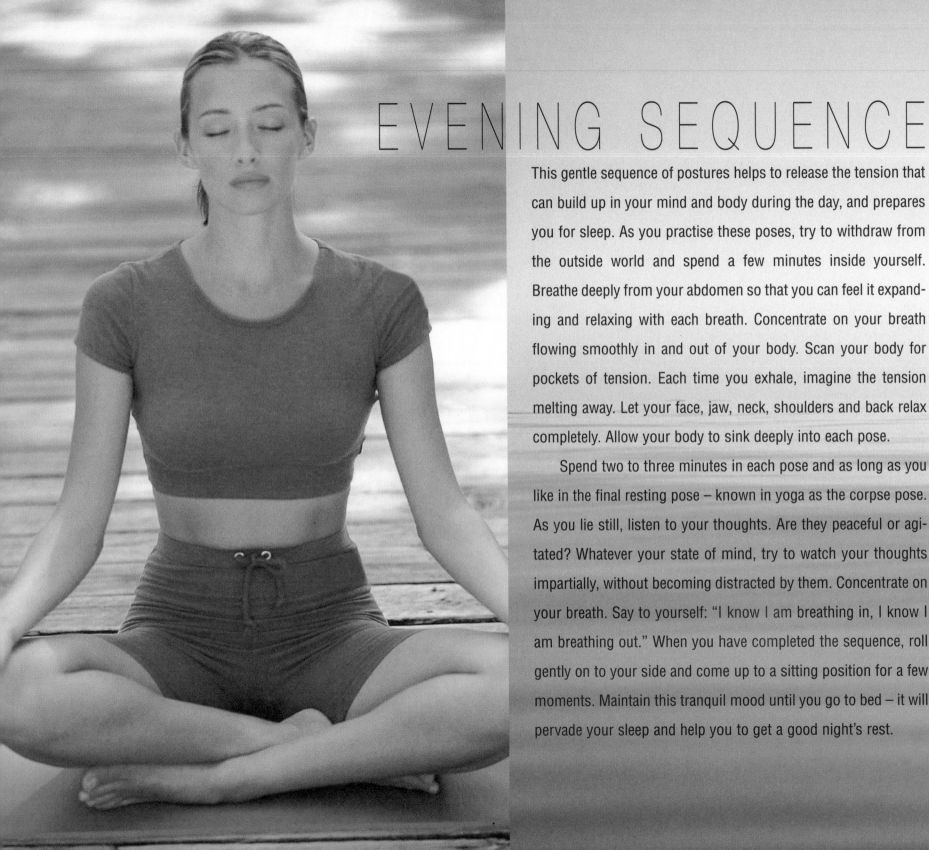

EVENING SEQUENCE

This gentle sequence of postures helps to release the tension that can build up in your mind and body during the day, and prepares you for sleep. As you practise these poses, try to withdraw from the outside world and spend a few minutes inside yourself. Breathe deeply from your abdomen so that you can feel it expanding and relaxing with each breath. Concentrate on your breath flowing smoothly in and out of your body. Scan your body for pockets of tension. Each time you exhale, imagine the tension melting away. Let your face, jaw, neck, shoulders and back relax completely. Allow your body to sink deeply into each pose.

Spend two to three minutes in each pose and as long as you like in the final resting pose – known in yoga as the corpse pose. As you lie still, listen to your thoughts. Are they peaceful or agitated? Whatever your state of mind, try to watch your thoughts impartially, without becoming distracted by them. Concentrate on your breath. Say to yourself: "I know I am breathing in, I know I am breathing out." When you have completed the sequence, roll gently on to your side and come up to a sitting position for a few moments. Maintain this tranquil mood until you go to bed – it will pervade your sleep and help you to get a good night's rest.

EVENING SEQUENCE

1 Lie flat on your back. Stretch your arms behind your head. Bring the soles of your feet together and let your knees fall outward.

2 Bring your knees in to your chest and hug them with your arms. Make small rocking movements from side to side.

3 Come back to centre and place your hands on your knees. Move your knees in circles (each knee in the opposite direction to the other). Start with small circles and slowly make them bigger. Now change directions.

4 Bring your knees back in to your chest and clasp them with your hands. Rock backward and forward in large movements so that you come on to your buttocks on the forward movements and on to your shoulder-blades during the backward movements. This helps to remove tension from the big muscles in your back.

5 Lie flat on your back with your legs a little way apart and your hands away from your body, palms facing up. Let your entire body sink into the floor. Close your eyes and focus on your breathing.

SEEK TRANQUILLITY

REST PEACEFULLY

ENJOY DEEP SLEEP

"The chariot of the mind is drawn by wild horses, and those wild horses have to be tamed." Svetasvatara Upanishad

REFLECTING UPON THE DAY

Over the course of the day, petty problems and minor irritations can build up so that by evening you almost feel overwhelmed by your worries. This can affect the quality of your sleep and may even keep you awake. If you are going to get a good night's rest, you need to clear your head of negative thoughts before bedtime. Imagine your mind is a sink full of dirty water. At the end of each day you must empty the sink and refill it with fresh, clean water. An effective way to achieve this mental cleansing exercise is to reflect on your day and then release your worries one by one.

CLEANSING THE MIND

Shortly before you go to bed, sit down in a quiet space where you can be alone with your thoughts. Imagine that your day has been a journey that started the moment you woke up. Now, mentally go back along the journey. Start with how you felt when you woke up this morning. Were you relaxed and rested or did you get up late and feel rushed and anxious? If you travelled to work, how was the journey? How did the rest of your day unfold? What obstacles did you face and how did you deal with them? How have you been feeling this evening? What kind of mood are you in now?

During this process of reflection you will probably find that your thoughts snag on stressful moments of your day and that you start replaying worrying events or, perhaps, upsetting remarks. Try to review these troubling moments constructively. Examine the cause of a problem, look at how you responded to it and then at what happened as a result of your behaviour. Psychologists call this the "ABC approach" – A is for "antecedent", B is for "behaviour" and C is for "consequence".

For example, suppose your train is late (antecedent); you get angry and argue with station staff (behaviour); this raises your stress levels so that when you finally get to work, you are snappy with co-workers and have difficulty concentrating (consequence). Now, focus on how you could have prevented this negative outcome by changing your behaviour. In this case, your train being late was beyond your control but you could have behaved differently by accepting the delay with equanimity and settling down to read a book or make notes for the day ahead.

Try to apply the ABC approach to all aspects of your day and, when you have done this, resolve to let each troubling event go. Imagine it floating away like a balloon in the sky – it appears to

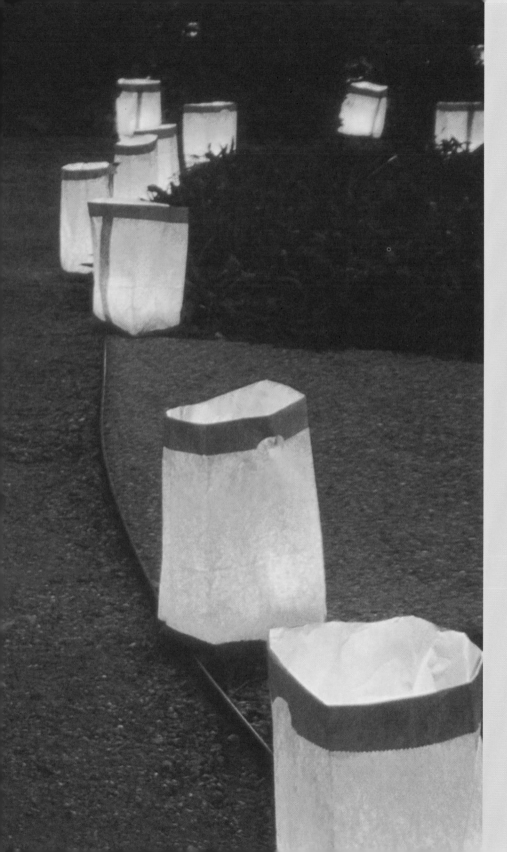

get smaller and smaller the higher it climbs until eventually it disappears from view. You can tackle persistent anxieties by writing them down in a list. If you need to take action to resolve a problem, write this down in a separate "to do" column. Now tell yourself that you have externalized the contents of your mind and that it is safe to let go of all the day's anxieties and truly relax.

Once you have finished reflecting upon the day in this way, bring your thoughts back to the present and remind yourself that you are sitting alone in a peaceful frame of mind. Rather than worrying about past or future events, try to be truly "present" in the moment. For example, focus on your breathing, look out of the window and lose yourself in the night sky, or concentrate on the sensation of your clothes – or bedclothes – against your skin.

End your reflections by saying a short prayer. A prayer does not have to be religious – it just contains a meaningful sentiment that you wish to express to yourself, much like the affirmations you might say at the start of the day (see page 14). For example, a prayer for self-acceptance might be: "Help me to accept those aspects about myself that I cannot change – so that I can devote all my energies to improving those things that I can change."

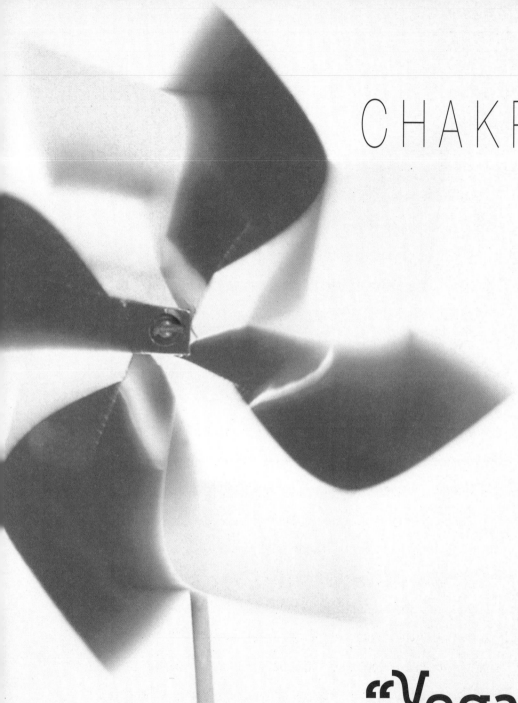

CHAKRA MEDITATION

In ancient Indian belief, the body is said to have seven energy centres, known as *chakras*. Meditating on the *chakras* at the end of the day helps to balance your energy and prepare your body for rest. Each *chakra* is located along a line running from your perineum to the crown of your head. The *chakras* are described as "spinning wheels of energy" and associated with certain colours, mantras and states of mental and spiritual awareness.

CHAKRA MEDITATION

To start, sit in a meditative posture (see pages 80–1) and breathe deeply. Concentrate on your root *chakra* (*muladhara*), on your perineum. As you inhale imagine you are drawing up red-coloured energy from the ground – feel a comforting sense of connection with the earth as you do this. As you exhale, imagine the energy spinning at your perineum and radiating outward. The

"Yoga is...a peace tha

root *chakra* governs physical needs. Meditating upon it eases muscular tension. Now, each time you inhale, imagine you are drawing the energy up to each *chakra* in turn (as described below) and seeing the energy change colour. Each time you exhale, visualize the energy spinning and glowing more strongly.

From the root *chakra*, imagine drawing the energy up to the spleen *chakra* (*swadhisthana*), in your abdomen. Visualize the energy changing to orange. This *chakra* is the centre of creativity and sexual energy. Meditating upon it brings release from egotism and sensual desires. Next, draw the energy up to the solar plexus *chakra* (*manipura*), just under the chest, where it changes to yellow. This *chakra* controls will and ambition. Meditating upon it strengthens willpower and self-control. Now visualize the energy flowing up to your heart *chakra* (*anahata*) and turning green. This *chakra* governs the emotions. Meditating upon it releases negative feelings such as anger and helps you cultivate love, empathy and compassion. Let the energy rise to your throat *chakra* (*vishuddi*) and turn blue. This chakra governs communication. Meditating upon it encourages self-expression and helps you to communicate with others.

Take the energy up to your third eye *chakra* (*ajna*), between your eyes, where it changes to indigo. This is the centre of intuition, insight and psychic power. Meditating upon it brings self-realization, inner wisdom and a deep sense of spiritual peace.

Draw the energy up to the crown *chakra* (*sahasrara*) on top of your head. See it turn violet. This *chakra* makes you at one with the universe. Imagine the energy becoming a golden light that radiates outward and envelopes your entire being. All the *chakras* are now balanced and spinning in vibrant vortices of pure energy. Keep breathing deeply and focus on feelings of bliss and peace.

is ever the same." The Bhagavad Gita

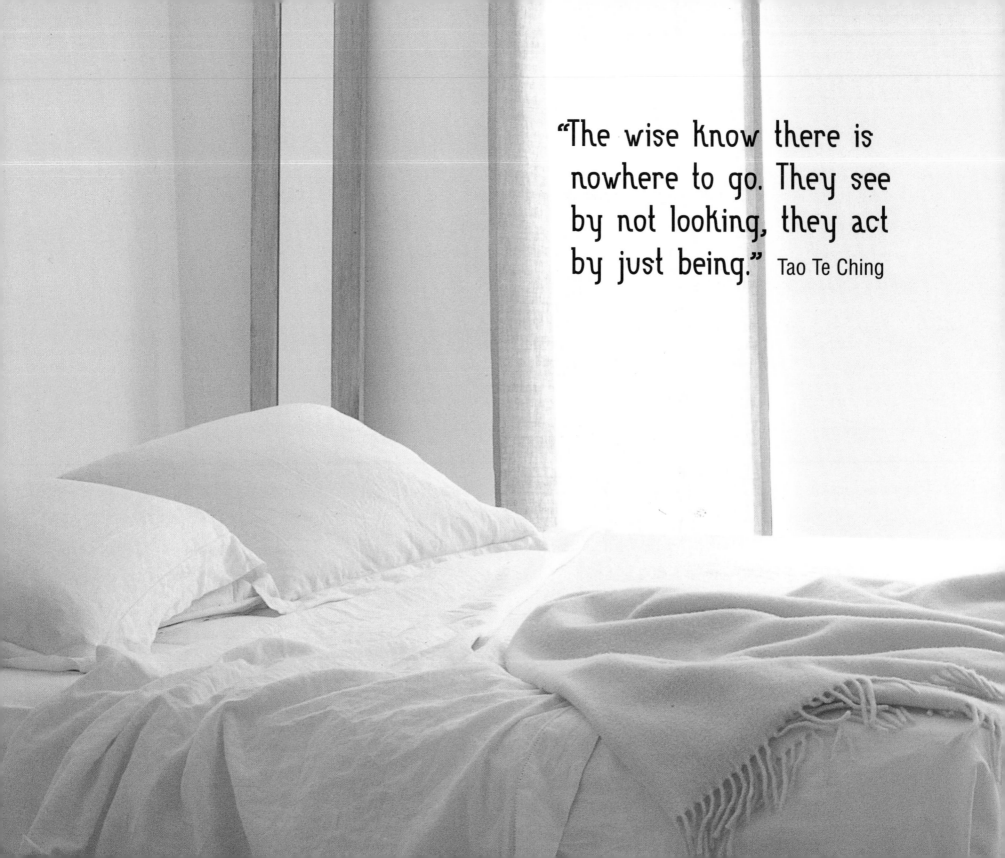

"The wise know there is nowhere to go. They see by not looking, they act by just being." Tao Te Ching

CREATING A HAVEN OF REST

Your sleeping place should be a sanctuary where you are assured of peace, privacy and security. The principles of feng shui – the Chinese art of object placement – can be applied to the bedroom as easily as your place of work (see page 38). For example, as with the workplace, feng shui experts believe the bedroom should be free of clutter. This allows *chi* energy to circulate while you sleep and recharge you for the day ahead. But, unlike a working environment, *chi* should not be too powerful or it may keep you awake. *Chi* is said to pass directly between the door and the window, so avoid positioning your bed directly between the two.

If your bed has space underneath it, feng shui practitioners recommend leaving this area clear to allow *chi* to flow freely. The bed should have a solid wooden headboard to protect your personal *chi* and recharge it while you rest. To help you feel more secure – and therefore more relaxed – feng shui masters say that the bed should be positioned so that you can see the door from where you lie, with the headboard close to a wall.

Symmetry is an important aspect of feng shui. Ideally, there should be space on both sides of the bed, and matching bedside tables and lamps. Mirrors, however, pose a problem in a bedroom as they are thought to drain your *chi* in your sleep. Avoid positioning a mirror where it can reflect your *chi* back at you where you lie. If possible, place the mirror on the inside of a wardrobe or cupboard door so you can shut it from view when not in use.

The best kind of bedroom is one that indulges your senses and generates feelings of emotional warmth and sensuality. Surround yourself with natural textures such as cotton, linen, silk, wool, mohair and cashmere. If you enjoy sleeping beneath lots of layers, cover the bed with shawls or throws that are tactile and sensual. Buy a good-quality non-synthetic mattress filled with natural fibres such as horsehair or coconut fibre and make sure it provides firm support for your spine.

Create the right mood by decorating your sleeping space in your favourite colours. Warm orange and terracotta are relaxing, rich reds stimulate passion, and blue is calming and soothing. You can also influence the mood of your sleeping space by using fragrant essential oils. Burn jasmine or ylang ylang oil to create an atmosphere of seduction, and rose, vanilla, camomile or lavender for relaxation. A bowl of fresh flowers or a sweet-smelling plant such as lavender are other ways to scent your sleeping space.

POSTURES FOR SLEEPING

Good posture is just as important when you are asleep as it is when you are sitting or standing. Adopting the correct posture for sleeping can go a long way to ensuring that you get a good night's rest and wake feeling refreshed. Sleep habits are deeply ingrained and it can be difficult to break old routines. If you want to change your sleeping posture, perhaps because you are waking up feeling stiff and aching, simply correct yourself each time you find yourself lying in your old posture. Eventually the new posture will feel so comfortable that your body will adopt it naturally.

According to some yoga writers, it is best to sleep on your side, as this encourages deep breathing through the nostrils, rather than shallow breathing through the mouth. Sleeping on your back can exaggerate the curve in the lower spine, leading to pain, especially in those suffering from back disorders. However, if you can only sleep on your back, by placing a firm pillow under your knees you can minimize the curve in the lower back and so avoid this problem. A common mistake is to have too many pillows. This throws the neck and spine out of alignment and can cause neck strain. Yoga experts recommend that you rest your head on a single firm pillow that is the depth of your shoulder.

The following sleeping positions are derived from yoga postures. The first, the prone posture, is best for taking a nap. Lie on your front with your head to one side, legs slightly apart and arms by your sides, a little way away from your body. (A variation of this posture is to raise your arms over your head – and fold them, if you need to, but avoid resting your head on your arms as this can reduce the circulation and cause tingling in your hands.)

The next two positions, the side relaxation pose (shown right) and the modified corpse pose, are suitable for sleeping all night. For the side relaxation pose, lie on your side with a pillow under your head to bring your head and spine into alignment. Bend your upper knee to form a right angle between your thigh and calf and rest the knee in front of you. (If you are pregnant or have a back disorder, place a pillow under this knee for comfort.) Bend your lower leg slightly. Rest your upper arm loosely across your diaphragm and stretch your lower arm out in front of you.

For the modified corpse pose, lie flat on your back with your legs a little way apart and your hands away from your body, palms facing up. Rest your head on a pillow to bring it into alignment with your spine and put a second pillow under your knees.

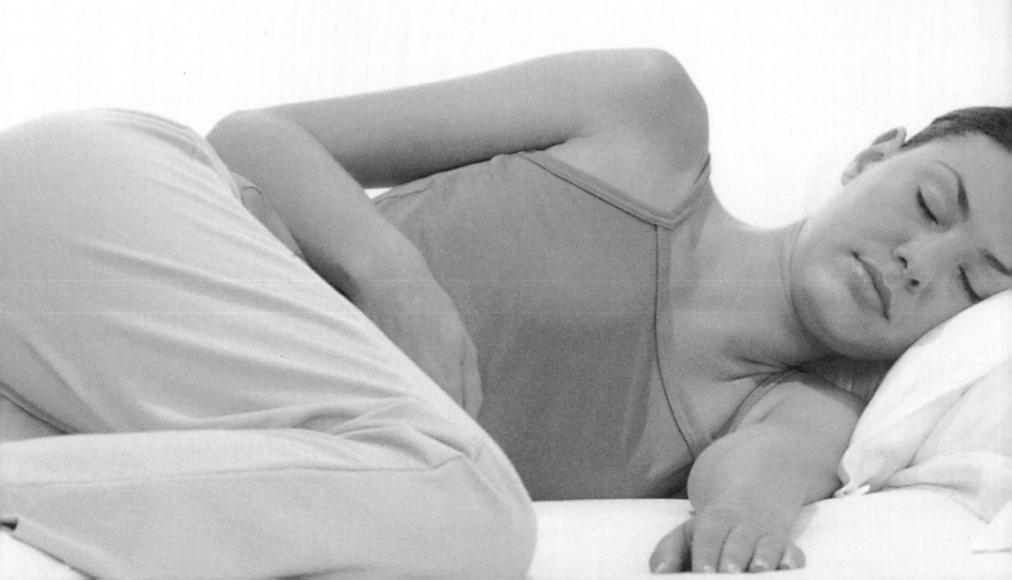

"The condition of deep sleep is one of oneness, a mass of silent consciousness made of peace and enjoying peace."

Mandukya Upanishad

VISUALIZATIONS FOR SLEEP

Despite everything you have done to get in a peaceful frame of mind, ready for sleep, you may find as you lie in bed that intrusive or repetitive thoughts keep you awake. The harder you strive to stop the flow of thoughts, the more elusive sleep becomes. One solution is to use visualization techniques to still your busy mind. Although visualization is often combined with other techniques, such as yoga, massage and meditation, it is also an effective method of quietening the mind when used on its own. All you need is your imagination. Simply picture a location that you find restful and soothing. This image, which could be a deserted beach or grassy bank beside a mountain stream, displaces your troublesome thoughts and induces a state of mental tranquillity.

Try to furnish your mental image with as much detail as possible so that you feel as if you are really there. For example, if you visualize a deserted beach, think about the colour of the sea and sand, the sound of the waves lapping against the shore, the quality of the light and the smells and sounds around you. How does the sand feel beneath your toes? If you look out to sea, what can you see on the horizon? Whatever you visualize, this is your special location – and you can return to it whenever you want.

CHOOSING A VISUALIZATION

Many people find quiet, natural views such as a woodland glade, a lake or a garden are particularly conducive to a restful state of mind. But you don't have to visualize a rural scene, your special place could just as easily be a church, a temple, a favourite room in a house or even a favourite chair in that room. You could choose a place from your past that you think of as being particularly beautiful or peaceful or one you associate with happy times.

There are other visualizations that you might find useful. For example, think of a sleeping cat or baby. Both breathe deeply and rhythmically as they sleep, enjoying total peace and relaxation. Imagine abandoning yourself to sleep in the same way. Visualize your body slowly turning to water and spreading out on the floor in a big pool, or think of a tranquil colour such as blue or green. Imagine it permeating your body with each breath you take.

BANISHING NEGATIVE THOUGHTS

Instead of displacing negative thoughts with positive images, you could visualize negative thoughts directly and imagine them dissipating. This is helpful when you are finding it difficult to hang

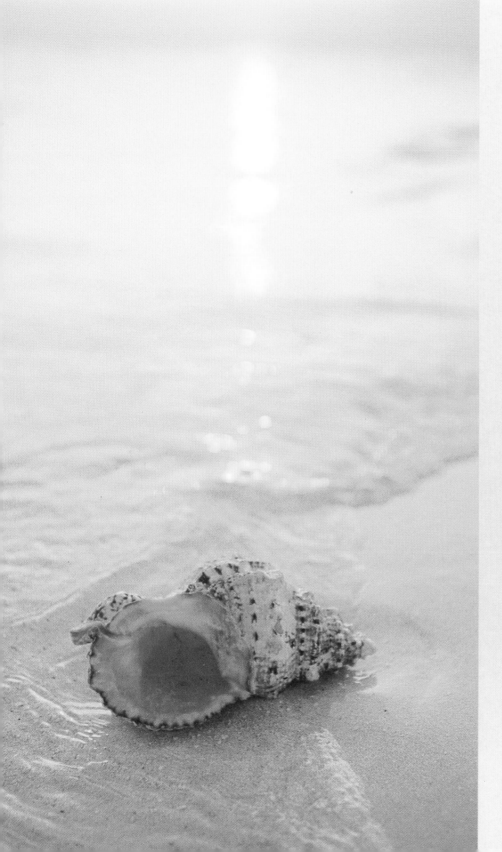

on to a positive mental image. For example, you could imagine that your thoughts are bubbles in a glass of fizzy lemonade. Watch them rise from the bottom of the glass to the top. Let them go as they burst into the open air. Imagine the bubbles are becoming fewer in number until the glass of lemonade becomes completely still. Alternatively, imagine that your thoughts are leaves being blown across your line of vision. Watch them blow past you in flurries; gradually imagine fewer leaves until they pass you one by one. Don't try to follow the leaves with your mind – just let them blow away.

If there is a specific problem you are trying to deal with, imagine you own a small box with a lock and key. Visualize the problem as a single tangible object – for example, a concern over a presentation at work might be represented by a marker pen. Take the object, and imagine placing it carefully inside the box. Visualize yourself closing the lid of the box and turning the key in the lock. Now imagine placing the box in a dark drawer. Tell yourself that you will retrieve it when you are ready to deal with the problem. If your thoughts drift back to the problem, imagine taking the box out of the drawer, giving it a shake and replacing it.

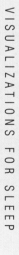

BIBLIOGRAPHY

FRASER, TARA *Yoga for You*, Duncan Baird Publishers, London (UK) and Thorsons, New York (US), 2001

FREKE, TIMOTHY (translator) *Tao Te Ching*, Piatkus, London (UK), 1995, and London Bridge, New York (US), 2000

GEORGE, MIKE *Learn to Relax*, Duncan Baird Publishers, London (UK) and Chronicle Books, San Francisco (US), 1998

GRIFFITHS, JAY *Pip Pip, A Sideways Look at Time*, HarperCollins, London (UK), 2000

HALL, MARI *Reiki*, Thorsons, London (UK) and New York (US), 2000

IYENGAR, B K S *Light on Pranayama*, Thorsons, London (UK) and New York (US), 1992

KORNFIELD, JACK *After the Ecstasy, the Laundry*, Rider Books, London (UK), 2000, and Bantam Doubleday Dell, New York (US), 2001

KRISHNAMURTI, JIDDU *Think on These Things*, HarperCollins, London and New York (US), 1997

LALVANI, VIMLA *Yoga for Sex*, Hamlyn, London (UK), 1999, and New York (US), 2001

LIVINGSTONE, ALISTAIR *Yoga for Energy*, Duncan Baird Publishers, London (UK), 2000

MASCARO, JUAN (translator) *The Bhagavad Gita*, Penguin, London (UK), 1962, and Viking Press, New York (US), 1983

MEHTA, NARENDRA *Indian Head Massage*, Thorsons, London (UK) and New York (US), 1999

MEHTA, SILVA, MIRA AND SHYAM *Yoga – the Iyengar Way*, Dorling Kindersley, London (UK), 1990, and Knopf, Maryland (US), 1990

MITCHELL, EMMA *Energy Exercises*, Duncan Baird Publishers, London (UK) and Tenspeed, Berkeley, CA (US), 2000

NHAT HANH, THICH *Present Moment Wonderful Moment*, Parallax Press, London (US) and Berkeley, CA (US), 1990

RINPOCHE, SOGYAL *The Tibetan Book of Living and Dying*, Rider Books, London (UK), 1992, and HarperCollins, San Francisco (US), 1994

ROWLEY, NIC AND HARTVIG, KIRSTEN *Energy Foods*, Duncan Baird Publishers, London (UK) and Tenspeed, Berkeley, CA (US), 2000

SCHIFFMAN, ERICH *Yoga, the Spirit and Practice of Moving into Stillness*, Pocket Books, New York (US) and Simon & Schuster, London (UK), 1997

SEKIDA, KATSUKI *Zen Training: Methods and Philosophy*, Weatherhill, New York (US), 1983

SMITH, KAREN *Massage: The Healing Power of Touch*, Duncan Baird Publishers, London (UK), 1998

VISHNU-DEVANANDA, SWAMI *Hatha Yoga Pradipika*, Lotus, New York (UK), 1997

WATTS, ALAN *Talking Zen*, Weatherhill, London (UK), New York (US) and Tokyo, 1994

WOOD, EARNEST *Seven Schools of Yoga*, Quest Books, Illinois (US), 1998

YOUNG, JACQUELINE *Acupressure for Health*, Thorsons, London (UK) and New York (US), 1994

INDEX

A

ABC APPROACH 150

ABDOMINAL BREATHING 84, 85

ACCEPTANCE 64

ACUPRESSURE 50–51

ACUPUNCTURE 22, 50

AFFIRMATIONS 14–15, 151

ALIGNMENT *SEE* POSTURE

ALLERGIES 48

ALTERNATE NOSTRIL BREATHING 46

ANXIETY 51

ARGUMENTS 133, 134

ATTACHMENT 132–3

ATTENTION *SEE* CONCENTRATION

ATTITUDES 14–15, 40–42, 61, 62–3

AWARENESS 10, 65, 89, 100–101, 151

B

BACK PAIN 50, 56, 59, 89

BALANCE 10, 52, 140

BALL OF ENERGY, QIGONG EXERCISES 24–5

BEDROOMS 155

BEING/DOING 68, 77

BOREDOM 41

BRAHMARI BREATH 144, 145

BREATHING 26–9, 38, 46, 48, 82–5

ALTERNATE NOSTRIL 46

BRAHMARI 144, 145

COMPLETE YOGA BREATH 26–7

DAN TIEN 23–4, 84

EXTENDING 85

MEDITATION 30, 42–3, 78, 82–5, 152

PARTNER 128, 136, 141

REIKI 48

DURING SLEEP 156

STRETCHES AND 16, 21, 24, 34, 59, 72–3, 89, 92–3, 146

T'AI CHI AND 20

BUCKWHEAT 104

BUDDHISM 30, 33, 40, 41, 64–6, 126

BEING/DOING AND 68, 77

LOVING KINDNESS AND 125, 126, 134

NATURE AND 77

NON-ATTACHMENT AND 132–3

SEE ALSO MINDFULNESS

C

CAFFEINE 120–21, 144

CALMING 30, 42–3, 46

CATEGORIZING 40–41

CENTRING 42–3

CEREMONY 121

CHAIRS 38

CHAKRAS 152–3

CHANGE 10–11

CHI SEE LIFE-FORCE ENERGY

CHILDREN 69, 118, 126

CHINESE MEDICINE 22, 50

CHINESE PHILOSOPHY 22–3

CLUTTER 38, 155

COLOUR 39, 155

COMPASSION 125, 126, 133

CONCENTRATION 30, 34, 41–3, 48, 65

COOKING 102, 106

SEE ALSO RECIPES

CORPSE POSE 89, 93, 144, 146, 156

CREATIVITY 66–7, 69

D

DAN TIEN 22–4, 84

DECISION-MAKING IN RELATIONSHIPS 139

DEHYDRATION 118

DESKS 38

DETOXIFICATION 110, 116

DIET *SEE* FOOD

DIGESTION 110, 119

DISCIPLINE 40, 41

DISTRACTIONS, LETTING GO OF 42–3

DIURETICS 120

DIZZINESS 8, 28, 84

DRINKS 98, 118–23, 144

E

EGO 64, 67, 133

EGYPTIAN POSE 44–5

ELIMINATION 110, 118, 119

EMOTIONAL RESPONSES 41, 134

ENERGY

CHANNELS 46

INCREASING 24, 25, 26–9, 39

SEE ALSO LIFE-FORCE ENERGY

ENLIGHTENMENT 33

ESSENTIAL OILS 39

E (continued)

EXERCISE 11, 52

FASTING AND 116

FLUID INTAKE AND 118

SLEEP AND 144

EXERCISES *SEE* STRETCHES; YOGA

EXPRESSION, ARTISTIC 66–7

EYES 48, 50, 56, 59, 77

F

FACIAL TENSION 56, 59, 89

FASTING 116–17

FATIGUE 51

FEAR 67, 132, 133

FENG SHUI 38, 155

FLAVOURINGS 102

FLOW 64, 66, 68

SEE ALSO UNDER LIFE-FORCE ENERGY

FLOWERS 38–9, 155

FLUIDS 98, 118–23

FOCUSING *SEE* CENTRING; CONCENTRATION

FOOD 97–109, 114–17, 122–3

SEE ALSO DRINKS

FOUNTAINS 39, 77

ACKNOWLEDGMENTS

Picture credits

The publishers would like to thank the following people and photographic libraries for permission to reproduce their material. Every care has been taken to trace copyright holders. However, if we have omitted anyone we apologize for this and will, if informed, make corrections in any future edition.

1 Photonica/Neo Vision 5 Mainstream/Ray Main 6 left Narratives/Jan Baldwin/Sophie Eadie 6 centre International Interiors/Paul Ryan (designer: Jacqueline Morabito) 6 right Telegraph Colour Library/Justin Pumfrey 7 left Telegraph Colour Library/Ericka McConnell 7 centre Stone/Jerome Ferraro 7 right Stone/James Darell 9 top left Matthew Ward/DBP 9 top right Mainstream/Ray Main 9 bottom left Mainstream/Ray Main 9 bottom right Photonica/Kazutomo Kawai 12 Narratives/Jan Baldwin/Sophie Eadie 13 Photonica/Kazutomo Kawai 14–15 Stone/Stephen Frink 16 Photonica/Neo Vision 16–19 Stone/Lorentz Gullachsen 17 Matthew Ward/DBP 20 Matthew Ward/DBP 21 Matthew Ward/DBP 22–23 Stone/Pierre Choiniere 24 IPC Syndication/David Brittain/Ideal Home 25 Matthew Ward/DBP 26–27 Stone/Reza Estakhrian 28 Matthew Ward/DBP 29 International Interiors/Paul Ryan (designer: Jacqueline Morabito) 31 Matthew Ward/DBP 32 International Interiors/Paul Ryan (designer: Jacqueline Morabito) 33 Photonica/Kaoru Mikami 34 Stone/Peter Nicholson 35 Matthew Ward/DBP 37 Stone/Colin Barker 39 Mainstream/Ray Main

40 Stone/Peter Dazeley 42–43 Mainstream/Ray Main (designer: Mick Allen) 43 left Matthew Ward/DBP 44 Matthew Ward/DBP 45 Matthew Ward/DBP 46 Matthew Ward/DBP 47 Matthew Ward/DBP 49 background Matthew Ward/DBP 49 left & right Matthew Ward/DBP 51 Matthew Ward/DBP 52 Photonica/Koutaku 53 Matthew Ward/DBP 55 Photonica/Johner 57 Matthew Ward/DBP 58 Matthew Ward/DBP 62–63 Photonica/S S Yamamoto 60 Telegraph Colour Library/Justin Pumfrey 61 Mainstream/Ray Main 65 Corbis/Charles & Josette Lenars 66 Stone/Jim Franco 69 Stone/Elie Bernager 72–73 Matthew Ward/DBP 75 Stone/Victoria Pearson 76 Mainstream/Ray Main 79 IPC Syndication/Peter Cassidy/Essentials 80 Matthew Ward/DBP 81 Matthew Ward/DBP 83 Matthew Ward/DBP 84 Mainstream/Ray Main 86 Matthew Ward/DBP 87 Matthew Ward/DBP 88–89 Stone/Robert Daly 92–3 Matthew Ward/DBP 95 Photonica/Neo Vision 96 Telegraph Colour Library/Ericka McConnell 97 Photonica/Masayoshi Hichiwa 99 Tim Winter 100 Stone/Amy Neunsinger 103 Sian Irvine/DBP 104 background Stone/Christel Rosenfeld 106 Photonica/Jane Yeomans 107 Sian Irvine/DBP 108 top Anthony Blake Photo Library/Tim Hill 108 bottom Stone/Chris Everard 110 William Lingwood/DBP 112 Matthew Ward/DBP 113 Photonica/Masayoshi Hichiwa 115 Sian Irvine/DBP 117 William Lingwood/DBP 118–119 William Lingwood/DBP 120 Stone/Victoria Pearson 123 bottom Image Bank/Antonio Rosario 123 top IPC

Syndication/Victoria Gomez 124 Stone/Jerome Ferraro 125 Mainstream/Ray Main 127 Mainstream/Ray Main 128 Photonica/Taniguchi 129 Matthew Ward/DBP 131 Matthew Ward/DBP 132 Stone/Stuart McClymont 134–135 Narratives/Polly Wreford 137 Matthew Ward/DBP 138 Matthew Ward/DBP 142 Stone/James Darell 143 International Interiors/Paul Ryan (designer: Jacqueline Morabito) 144 Stone/Simon Battensby 145 Mainstream/Ray Main 146 Camera Press/Shaz 147 Matthew Ward/DBP 156–157 Matthew Ward/DBP 149 Photonica/Magnus Rietz 151 Corbis/Richard Cummins 152 Image Bank/M Tcherevkoff 154 International Interiors/Paul Ryan (designer: Jacqueline Morabito) 158–159 Stone/Pete Seaward

Publishers' acknowledgments:

Design assistance: Suzanne Tuhrim

Hair and make-up: Dawn Lane

Models: Estelle Jaumotte and Jason Bailey (MOT)